PRIVATE PRACTICE MANAGEMENT
in Physical Therapy

PRIVATE PRACTICE MANAGEMENT
in Physical Therapy

Ira M. Fiebert, Ph.D., P.T.

Adjunct Associate Professor
Division of Physical Therapy
Department of Orthopaedics and Rehabilitation
University of Miami School of Medicine
Miami, Florida
Co-owner, Physical Therapy Associates, P.A.
Miami, Florida
Co-owner, Physical Therapy Institute, Inc.
Delray Beach, Florida

Linda J. Zane, M.P.A., P.T.

Co-owner and President, Physical Therapy Institute, Inc.
Delray Beach, Florida

Eileen F. Hamby, M.B.A., P.T.

President, Health Management Specialists, Inc.
Hollywood, Florida

Churchill Livingstone
New York, Edinburgh, London, Melbourne

Library of Congress Cataloging-in-Publication Data

Fiebert, Ira M.
    Private practice management in physical therapy / by Ira M. Fiebert,
Linda J. Zane, Eileen F. Hamby.
      p. cm.
    Includes bibliographical references.
    ISBN 0-443-08618-4
    1. Physical therapy—Practice. 2. Small business—Management.
I. Zane, Linda J. II. Hamby, Eileen F. III. Title.
    [DNLM: 1. Physical Therapy. 2. Practice Management, Medical.
3. Private Practice—organization & administration. WB 460 F452p]
RM713.F53   1990
615.8'2'0068—dc20
DNLM/DLC
for Library of Congress   89-71196
                                             CIP

Distributed in the United Kingdom by Churchill Livingstone, Robert Stevenson House, 1–3 Baxter's Place, Leith Walk, Edinburgh EH1 3AF, and by associated companies, branches, and representatives throughout the world.

Acquisitions Editor: *Kim Loretucci*
Copy Editor: *Elizabeth Bowman*
Production Designer: *Jill Little*
Production Supervisor: *Christina Hippeli*

Printed in the United States of America

First published in 1990

In memory of my father,
Richard Fiebert

Preface

Physical therapists have several arenas in which to provide patient care. Some may opt, for reasons of autonomy, to open private practices. What they will discover, either at the onset or further down the road, is that their education has not prepared them for the business aspects of a practice, which require so many diverse skills to run successfully.

The purpose of this book is to provide guidelines for opening and running a private practice. The first portion of the book covers the start-up issues and the second portion discusses the day-to-day management of the private practice.

One component of initiating a practice is the self-assessment of personal attributes, philosophy, and goals; the first portion of the book discusses this component and provides guidelines for identifying personal strengths and weaknesses. Also discussed is the variety of practice alternatives (e.g., partnership, corporation) from which the new practitioner may choose. The requirements for initial funding and the roles played by support systems are discussed, along with deciding upon the location of the practice and the design of the physical facility.

The second half of the book will aid the new practitioner after the practice is up and running. It discusses the development of policies and procedures, the day-to-day responsibilities of various personnel, the maintenance of a budget, and the critical issues of marketing and of developing a referral base. A guideline for financial reimbursement, which can sometimes be burdensome, is provided. Assuming the private practice is a success, this book concludes with future possibilities for growth and expansion.

Thus, in a step-by-step fashion, the book guides the reader through the process of initiating and managing a private practice. Hopefully the physical therapist contemplating such a move will consult this book first. For those who have already made the jump and are enjoying the fruits of their labor, this book should provide some helpful insights to enhance the future of their practice.

Ira M. Fiebert
Linda J. Zane
Eileen F. Hamby

Contents

1

PERSONAL SKILLS AND PROFESSIONAL PHILOSOPHY AND GOALS

When physical therapists enter private practice, to be successful they must also become executive managers and businesspeople. This requires them to develop skills in areas foreign to their clinical expertise. In many instances the physical therapist is not fully prepared for the demands of starting and managing a private practice; however, a thorough self-assessment when contemplating such a move helps to determine strengths and weaknesses.

PERSONAL SKILLS
Physical Therapy Management

Of course, clinical skill is of utmost importance in providing quality health care to patients. All potential private practitioners must honestly assess their clinical abilities. Experience in treating certain types of patients must be identified, as must the situations in which the practitioner is relatively inexperienced. Making up any deficits may be necessary to remain competitive in the patient care market.

Administration

Most physical therapists are deficient in administrative skills as a result of minimal training in administration during their formal education. Therefore, would-be private practitioners should explore different administrative styles and determine the most effective approach for them.

Communication Skills

Ability to communicate successfully with referring physicians, patients, health care providers, insurance providers, and employees will greatly enhance success in private practice. Physical therapists, like all individuals, will vary greatly in their abilities to communicate effectively.

Business Aptitude

An excellent clinician can fail in private practice if he or she is not prepared for the business end of the practice. Necessary business skills include the ability to negotiate, purchase, sell, bill, collect, and manage, among many others.

Aesthetic Sensibilities

Aesthetic decisions make a formal statement about the practice, determining the manner in which it is presented to others. The business card, brochure, office furnishing, and dress code are a few of the items that fall under the category of aesthetics (see Ch. 10). Physical therapists receive no formal training in aesthetics; therefore, this skill is a uniquely individualized one.

Assessing Present Level of Skills

When the time to start the private practice arrives, physical therapists must be cognizant of their knowledge and skills in the above areas. An honest assessment of these skills will prove valuable in selecting partners and employees with complementary skills, thereby strengthening the practice. Accordingly, practitioners who have thoroughly identified their strengths and weaknesses will be able to develop a realistic business plan.

PERSONAL SKILLS CHECKLIST

Level of Skill:	Low	Average	High
Clinical skills	_____	_____	_____
Administrative skills	_____	_____	_____
Communication skills	_____	_____	_____
Business skills	_____	_____	_____
Aesthetic skills	_____	_____	_____

DEVELOPMENT OF A PROFESSIONAL PHILOSOPHY

The development of a professional philosophy varies from one professional practitioner to another. A philosophy is based upon an individual's values—that is, beliefs about the way things should be. Various experiences throughout life shape the development of a person's value base. Eventually, through individual maturation, people develop internally consistent value systems by which they make decisions, both personal and professional. Observations and experiences from prior employment and professional situations enable them to develop a professional value base consistent with their personal value base. This professional value base is reflected in the philosophy of the private practice.

DEVELOPMENT OF PROFESSIONAL GOALS

Goals are measurable outcomes that the private practice may achieve by a specified point in time. These goals must represent the practice's philosophy. The goals developed for a private practice are used objectively to set action plans and evaluate the productivity of the methodologies employed. Some areas of goal setting for private practices are: quality of care, delivery of service, management style, and marketing strategy.

Quality of Care

Quality of care is an abstract concept largely determined by the practice's philosophy. The definition of quality of care is based on values that individual professionals must choose for themselves. The amount of time spent by physical therapists with patients, the amount of advanced training that they have in specialized areas, the utilization of support personnel, and the amount of sophisticated equipment on hand all play a role in determining the practice's definition of quality of care.

Goals related to quality of care may pertain to patients' complaints or lack of complaints. The cultivating of new referral sources may reflect quality of care.

Delivery of Services

Delivery of services affects quality of care. The range of options pertaining to delivery of services is broad. At one extreme physical therapy services are delivered solely by licensed physical therapists, while at the other extreme such services are provided by unlicensed persons. The use or overuse of untrained individuals to deliver services, although highly remunerative in the short term, could seriously damage the reputation of the practice in the long term. The choice of who provides physical therapy services reflects the quality-of-care philosophy of the owner(s) of the practice.

The frequent use of highly reimbursable procedures also can generate considerable revenue, and the use of unlicensed personnel to apply these procedures considerably decreases the operating costs of the practice. Another important question is how long a patient should continue with physical therapy if objective improvement is not noted; a long-term patient increases revenues. Therefore, when developing goals concerning delivery of services, the practitioners must assess their professional philosophy.

Management Style

There are two primary management styles of private practice, based largely on concern for service versus concern for workers. The former approach is centered around the belief that the service provided, in this instance patient care, is of primary importance. The concern for staff is centered around the belief that the needs of the therapists, assistants, aides, and office personnel are of primary importance.

The concern for service leads the therapist to strive for efficiency of task performance. In private practice this means meeting patient needs, which include convenience of scheduling, minimal time in the waiting room, expedient treatment, appropriate verbal and written communication, and any other conditions that affect the quality of patient services.

Concern for workers centers on thoughtful attention to the staff's needs. In private practice this means providing a friendly, comfortable work environment, including appropriate scheduling of patients, fair work hours, adequate work area, necessary equipment, and an appropriate fringe benefit package.

There are various degrees of compromise between concern for service and concern for workers. The worst scenario occurs when management shows minimal concern for both service and workers, which in private practice means that the owner(s) provides minimum services for both patients and staff. A practice with only one therapist working extended hours in one treatment cubicle would represent this type of situation. In the best scenario management provides an environment for motivated workers who have a vested interest in the organization and work for its goals. In private practice this would mean specialized therapists who work interdependently in a comfortable, fully equipped office with the necessary support personnel.

Once again, it becomes apparent that in developing the private practice the philosophy of the owner influences all decisions. Goals related to service may relate to the number of treatments provided or the types of diagnoses for which patients are treated in the facility. Goals related to workers may relate to the development by therapists of specialized clinical skills, their achievement of advanced academic degrees, or their active involvement in their professional association.

Marketing Strategy

Marketing is the art and science of assessing what is needed to promote the practice and then meeting that need. When marketing the private practice, the methods chosen are derived from the philosophy and goals of the practice.

If the marketing techniques used inform physicians, insurance carriers, and the public that the practice provides services by licensed physical therapists only, then only licensed physical therapists may be used; if the strategy is to inform these groups that the practice provides quality care at a lower price than the local hospital, then the fee schedule has to support this claim. If the marketing approach informs consumers that they do not have to wait longer than 15 minutes to receive their therapy, the scheduling pattern must ensure this (see Chapter 10).

It is also obvious that marketing strategies must reflect the philosophy and goals of the private practice. Essentially these strategies are derived from the values of the practice's owner(s), through which they are able to develop plans and implement strategies for operating as part of the health care community.

PROFESSIONAL VALUES CHECKLIST

The physical therapist contemplating private practice should identify professional values as they relate to the following four entities:

Quality of care   _____

Delivery of services   _____

Management style   _____

Marketing considerations   _____

SUMMARY

This chapter has discussed the areas of physical therapy clinical skills, administration, communication, and business management aesthetics, in relation to private physical therapy practice. The honest identification of assets and liabilities pertaining to each area is critical for the development of a successful practice. The philosophy and goals of a physical therapy practice have been addressed as they relate to quality of care, delivery of services, management style, and marketing considerations.

SUGGESTED READINGS

Barnes M, Crutchfield C: Job satisfaction-dissatisfaction: A comparison of private practitioners and organizational physical therapists. Phys Ther 57(1):35–41, 1977

Blake R, Mouton J: The Managerial Grid. Gulf Publishing, Houston, 1964

Burch EA, Inglarsh A: A conversation about starting a private practice. Phys Ther Today 11(4):37–42, 1988

Fiebert IM, Barbe R: Private practitioners ARE different. Whirlpool 6(2):14–16, 1983

Grannis C: Advantages and disadvantages of private practice therapy. Whirlpool 2(3):2–9, 1979

Peters TJ, Waterman RH Jr: In Search of Excellence. Warner Books, New York, 1982

Profile of a private practice physical therapist—Results of the PPS survey. Whirlpool: 8(2):26–29, Summer 1985

2

TYPES OF PRIVATE PRACTICE

There are many ways for physical therapists to enter private practice, of which some entail major and others only minimal financial investment.

The considerable capital invested in developing and opening an office varies with the size of the facility, number of owners, target population, and capital assets available. The private office environment will be addressed in the following discussions of sole practice and group practice.

Alternate forms of private practice that do not require large financial investments are available to physical therapists. The costs are considerably reduced when office overhead and major pieces of equipment are not necessary. Alternative environments that will be considered include joint ventures, contract therapy, home health care, private practice employee status, and public schools.

WAYS TO SET UP A PRIVATE PRACTICE
Sole Practice

Those physical therapists who wish to "go it alone" are considered sole practitioners. They are willing to assume responsibility for all phases of their private practice. They enjoy the power—and, they hope, the glory—associated with sole responsibility for all decisions and the outcomes of their decisions.

However, the sole practitioner will have an immense amount of work to do before opening the office and will need to make a considerable commitment of time and energy. Even if the therapist is extremely well organized, all the activities that rely on outside persons—landlords, vendors, graphic designers, lawyers, accountants, architects, and contractors—take considerable time and require emotional fortitude on the part of the practitioner, who must deal with all outside people and their associated agencies or companies. Usually, new private practitioners assume that the outside sources will deliver their services on the stated deadline and will meet the standard of quality clearly understood by all. However, this may never happen. After they have been paid, either on account or in full, the outside service persons may become lax about deadlines and even about performing quality work. Problems do arise and must be dealt with by the sole practitioner.

There are both benefits and drawbacks to a sole practice. All decisions, including those about location, lease, floor plan, support personnel, purchases, and employees, must be made by the practitioner alone. The fact that the sole practitioner can react and decide rapidly is a positive factor, but the rapidity of response and the lack of input from others may lead to incorrect decisons, which can prove detrimental to the practice.

The most significant benefit of starting a private practice alone is the fact that the sole practitioner reaps all the rewards if the practice is successful. The tangible forms of the rewards (cash, life insurance, annuities, automobiles, etc.) once again are determined by the practitioner alone.

Group Practice

Whereas the sole practitioner assumes responsibility for all aspects of the new practice, the members of a group practice share the responsibilities, thereby decreasing the time commitment of the individual group members, each of whom is responsible for only a percentage of the required activities. Moreover, the activities can be divided according to which members have the most skill for specific required tasks. Thus, the group member with some knowledge about designing a physical therapy facility may deal with the architects and construction people; the member with the best public relations skills may coordinate marketing activities; and the member with legal and accounting skills may deal with the lawyer and the accountant. This method of sharing the work load is one of the major benefits of group practice.

Even with sharing of activities, most members of group private practices still desire input on all decisions. Therefore, a member assigned a specific task will have to report back to the others prior to a group decision and resulting implementation. This obviously can create delays both in the decision process and in implementaton and can also create difficulty among group members when agreement is not attainable. On the other hand, this type of process frequently can produce more sophisticated decisions and prevent major and costly errors.

The most significant disadvantage of group practice is that the potential rewards of success must be shared among the group members. If the practice is financially successful, all the members of the group are entitled to share in the benefits. Once again, the joint decision making process must be used to determine the best way in which to share the benefits of the practice. As a result of individual differences, *compromise* becomes a key word.

Sole versus Group Practice

When trying to decide between a sole and a group practice, practitioners must consider their own professional and personal assets. If a sole practice is chosen, the practitioner must possess the necessary clinical, administrative, and com-

Table 2-1. Comparison between Sole and Group Practice

	Sole Practice	Group Practice
Clinical skills	Solo	Shared
Administrative skills	Solo	Shared
Communication skills	Solo	Shared
Work load	Solo	Shared
Financial obligation	Solo	Shared

munication skills. For practitioners who do not believe that they have these skills to the necessary degree, a group arrangement may permit them to enter private practice successfully by selecting associates with complementary skills. In a sole practice the total work-related responsibility rests solely on the practitioner; in a group practice work responsibilities can be shared. Another critical factor to consider in deciding between a sole and a group practice is the initial financial obligation. If this is too high for the individual, a group endeavor may become necessary in order to share financial obligation. Table 2-1 compares sole with group practice.

LEGAL STRUCTURES FOR PRIVATE PRACTICES

There are many structural varieties of private practice in the United States. In developing a practice the various structures must be considered and the best alternative for each situation chosen.

Sole Proprietorship

A business owned and operated by one person is a sole proprietorship. Such a business is easy to organize and start up, as it usually does not require special government permission to operate or special legal documentation among co-owners. Essentially, one starts to work for oneself and thereby becomes a sole proprietor.

A sole proprietorship exists as long as the owner maintains the practice. Accordingly, it is easy to open and close this type of practice. The fact that all decisions are made by one person makes for simplicity in operation as well. Managerial methods are determined by the individual owner, who can rapidly alter managerial philosophy when necessary. In this type of practice there are few government regulations aside from paying taxes. All taxes are considered to be owed by the individual owner, and therefore this arrangement may serve as a tax advantage.

On the other hand, there are some disadvantages to sole proprietorship, the major one being the owner's unlimited liability for all financial obligations incurred. If the practice is unable to meet these obligations, the practitioner's individual and private, non-business-related assets may be attached to cover the business liabilities.

An additional disadvantage is that the practice is limited by the individual limitations of the practitioner. Raising capital may be a problem as the only security a financial institution could obtain would consist of the proprietor's assets. If the practitioner receives a salary from the business, then the collateral for the finances may be placed at risk. If the practice is small, it may not offer growth potential for employees, and therefore attracting and keeping quality employees will be a problem.

Partnership

A business owned and operated by more than one individual is a partnership. The minimum number of individuals for a partnership is two, and the maximum number is unlimited. A partnership must have an agreement between the partners, and this should be handled by attorneys.

A partnership is a cooperative effort between individuals whereby sharing of responsibilities and collaboration in the use of skills can prove to be assets. The partnership agreement must address many avenues of concern, which include the responsibilities of each partner, salaries, benefits, the buy-sell agreement, the decision making process, and handling of profits.

The advantages of choosing a partnership are multifold. A partnership can continue to exist in the event that one of the owners no longer wishes or is no longer able to remain in the business. Increased knowledge and skills are available that should facilitate solid decision making and management. The ability to grow and expand is increased over that of a sole proprietorship, since there are more owners, each of whom can oversee various endeavors. With the assets of more than one owner available for collateral, the potential for obtaining financing is clearly increased. All taxes are considered part of the individual owners' obligations, and this may serve as a tax advantage.

On the other hand, there are some disadvantages to partnerships, the major one being that all partners have unlimited liability. This means that each partner is responsible for all financial obligations incurred by the practice. Worse yet, each of the partners has the right, on behalf of the partnership, to enter into agreements for which all partners are fully obligated. If an obligation exists, the creditors can demand payment from all or only one of the partners. The partners' non-business-related assets are subject to attachment to cover the business liabilities.

An additional disadvantage is that the partnership can develop internal friction if the various partners have significantly different ideas and philosophies. It may also prove difficult for one partner to leave the partnership if the others wish to continue.

When considering the concept of partnership, two terms frequently used are *general partners* and *limited partners*. General partners are those, discussed above, who have unlimited liability and have the right to manage the partnership. Limited partners are partners who invest in the practice and are only responsible to the extent of their investment. They have neither unlimited liability nor the right to manage the business.

Corporation

A corporation is essentially an artificial person or a legal entity that conducts business in its own name. Through incorporation, practitioners can enter private practice jointly or alone. Since a corporation is a legal entity, effort is required to create one. The development of a legal corporation entails a corporate name search within the charter state, the filing of legal documents with state and local government, and the payment of fees. Additionally, corporations maintain corporate kits, stock certificates, a corporate seal, and minutes of corporate meetings. Corporate by-laws must be developed to spell out management procedures (see Ch. 4). Retention of legal counsel is essential when incorporating a private practice.

The owners of a corporation are known as *stockholders* or *shareholders* and receive proof of ownership in stock certificates. There are two types of stockholders, common and preferred. The former have the right to vote at stockholder meetings; the latter do not normally vote at meetings but receive their share of profits before the common stockholders. The stockholders elect the board of directors, which is empowered to manage the corporation. The board of directors selects the officers of the corporation, usually a president, vice-president(s), treasurer, and secretary. These officers have the right to make commitments on behalf of the corporation.

In many instances the stockholders and the board of directors are the same persons, namely the private practitioners. However, in large, multistate corporations there will be many stockholders in addition to the directors. When the stockholders and the board of directors are one and the same, the corporation operates similarly to a partnership. Agreements between the stockholders need to be spelled out with respect to the responsibilities of each owner, salaries, benefits, the buy-sell agreement, the decision making process, handling of profits, etc.

Like a partnership, a corporation can continue to exist when one of the owners no longer wishes or is no longer able to continue in the business. Having more than one owner increases the knowledge and skills base, which should facilitate solid decision making and management. A further advantage for the corporation is the ability to raise additional capital, if needed, through the issuance of stock. Usually, a new corporation issues only a percentage of its authorized stock to the owners. This allows for the sale of additional stock at a later date. The stockholders vote in accordance with the proportion of stock they own. The

Table 2-2. Comparison of Private Practice Structural Entities

	Sole Practitioner	Partnership	Corporation
Organizing	Easy	Some difficulty	Most difficulty
Responsibility	Total	Shared	Shared
Financial obligation	All	Shared	Shared
Legal needs	Some	Some	Considerable
Government intervention	Minimal	Minimal	Some
Ability to change	Fast	Slow	Slow
Expansion potential	Limited	Greater	Greatest
Benefits	All	Shared	Shared
Liabilities	Unlimited	Unlimited	Limited

ability of the corporation to sell stock is a method of expanding and financing the business. The ability of the individual owners to sell their respective shares of stock provides a method of leaving the practice while the practice continues to function.

The major advantage of an incorporated private practice over a partnership is that the owners have limited liability. A corporation, as a separate and legal entity, obligates the shareholders only to the extent of their involvement. Personal assets are not liable for covering the corporation's obligations. The ability to grow, expand, and raise capital are all greater for a corporation than for the business structures discussed previously.

On the other hand, there are some disadvantages to incorporation. Corporations are taxed at a higher rate than individuals. Accordingly, the corporation will pay higher taxes than the partnership. However, there is a type of corporation, the Subchapter S option, that allows the stockholders to be taxed directly. They thereby benefit from the lower taxers they would pay in a partnership while retaining the benefits of incorporation. However, private practitioners should communicate with their accountant before deciding whether the Subchapter S option is best for their particular practice.

Further disadvantages of incorporating a private practice: an incorporated private practice is subject to all government rules and regulations that apply to corporations, and start-up and operating costs are greater for corporations than for sole proprietorships and partnerships.

Three formal structures for private practice have been described—the sole proprietorship, the partnership and the corporation. In Table 2-2 these structures are compared with respect to nine important features.

Additional Ways to Enter Private Practice

Joint Venture

A joint venture can be considered a synergistic relationship between two or more components of a business project. The concept of joint ventures has gained momentum in the health community during the late 1980s. Hospitals are forming joint ventures with physician groups, corporations with health care providers, and physicians with physical therapists, to name a few examples.

The appeal of joint ventures for physical therapists is that by undertaking one with a group of physicians, they ensure a base of patient referrals. The project can be set up as a corporation with the various groups owning shares of stock and thereby having limited liability.

The concern for physical therapists has to be with the actual control over the physical therapy domain. The group that holds the greater number of stock shares controls the joint venture. If private physical therapy practitioners enter into joint ventures with physicians, it is imperative for them to have legal counsel to represent their interests and to elaborate on the business arrangement.

Contract Arrangements

Contract therapy can be arranged on two levels. On the first level an entrepreneur sets up a business and hires physical therapists to provide services to various facilities on a contract basis. On the second level a private practitioner works on a contract basis for himself or herself.

When starting a business in which therapists will provide contract services, the private practitioner can set it up as a sole proprietorship, a partnership, or a corporation. The aim of this business is to find facilities that require physical therapy services but are usually unable to fill their full-time physical therapy positions and therefore have to contract for weeks or months at a time for such services. In addition to finding facilities that require services, the contract business also must find physical therapists who are willing to provide their services on a short-term basis. The business profits by charging the facilities a higher dollar amount per hour of service than it pays its contract therapists.

Private practitioners who provide contract therapy are essentially working as sole practitioners. They are able to accept or reject contract work as they see fit, thereby controlling their work schedule. The other benefit to this type of private practice is that the pay scale for contract therapy is considerably higher than the hourly wage of therapists on a facility's payroll. The down side of this type of practice occurs when less contract work is available than the practitioner wishes to undertake. However, this version of contract therapy provides many of the benefits of private practice without a major financial undertaking.

Home Health Care

Another form of private practice is provision of care in patients' homes. This type of practice also has two levels—the therapist either may work as a sole proprietor, receiving payment for each visit, as does the contract therapist, or may work as a full- or part-time employee of a home health care agency.

Employee

An inexpensive way to prepare for private practice is to first work as an employee for a private service, which may be office-based, a contracting facility, or a home health care agency. Working as an employee guarantees the therapist

Table 2-3. Comparisons of Various Methods of Private Practice

Type	Location	Responsibility	Expense	Potential Revenues
Sole practice	Clinic	All	All	Unlimited
Group practice	Clinic	Shared	High shared	Unlimited shared
Joint venture	Clinic	Varies	Varies	Varies
Contract				
Others	Office	All	Low	Unlimited
Self	Varies	All	None	Limited (by the amount one person can generate)
Home health care	Homes	All	None	Limited (by the amount one person can generate)
Employee	Clinic	None	None	Limited
Public school	Schools	All	None	Limited

a salary, benefits, and suitable working conditions without any of the risks associated with private practice. It also provides a training ground for a future plunge as the owner of a private practice.

Public Schools

The public schools in many cities provide physical therapy services by employing their own therapists, contracting services to companies or individuals, or a combination of both. Depending upon what is available in various cities, private practitioners have the opportunity to offer contract services on either of the previously mentioned levels or to work as an employee in the public schools.

SUMMARY

This chapter discusses the many avenues that physical therapists have available to them to enter private practice. These paths vary in the magnitude of risk therapists assume, the work location, the type of patients treated, and the possibilities for growth and expansion. Since many paths exist, it is most likely that physical therapists seeking to enter private practice will be able to find one that meets their needs (Table 2-3).

SUGGESTED READINGS

Johnston BE, Lord PJ: Your Private Practice "Planning and Organization." Ben E. Johnston Jr. & Peter J Lord, Lake City, FL, 1982

J.K. Lasser Tax Institute: How to Run a Small Business. 6th Ed. McGraw-Hill, New York, 1989

Shilling D: Be Your Own Boss—The Complete, Indispensible, Hands-on Guide to Starting and Running Your Own Business. Penguin Books, New York, 1983

Snook ID, Kaye EM: A Guide to Health Care Joint Ventures. Aspen Publishers, Rockville, MD, 1987

Straub JT, Kossen S: Introduction to Business. PWS—KENT Publishing, Boston MA, 1983

3

INITIAL FUNDING

SOURCES OF FUNDING

After deciding to enter private practice, the practitioner must assess the practicality of the venture. A very critical issue is where to obtain the funds to undertake this task.

Initial funding may come from many sources. Two primary sources are personal assets and money borrowed from lending establishments. Either method entails variables that directly affect the physical therapist both personally and as part of the business.

The Practitioner's Own Money

When trying to secure capital dollars for a new business, physical therapists must expect to use some of their own money. The question is how much or what percentage of the financing this should be. Lending institutions take the approach that if the borrowers are not willing to risk some of their own money, there is no reason for the lending institution to risk its money.

A physical therapist may be able to provide some capital from personal savings. If the therapist does not have savings, family members may lend some money to facilitate the new business effort. If neither of these alternatives is viable, the therapist may be able to take out a second home mortgage, thus borrowing against the worth of the home. Another alternative would be to sell possessions to raise the necessary capital.

It is imperative to remember the benefit of financing with other people's money (i.e., it is better to borrow money for the business than to tie up one's own). This approach is best when interest rates are low. When interest rates are inflated, the amount one must pay on the borrowed money makes loan repayment more difficult.

The advantage of using other people's money is that one still has access to one's own funds for personal use. Investing all one's money in a business may leave one with insufficient funds for personal needs. If the money is not tied up in the business, the business may be struggling, but the owner and the owner's family retain access to personal assets for enjoyment, education, or an emergency.

A Partner's Money

One method of using other people's money is to form a partnership or corporation. These alternatives require initial funding from more than one person. The percentage and actual dollar amounts of each person's investment, but also that person's share of ownership and control over the practice, are thereby decreased (see Ch. 2). If one enters private practice with other people, the same problem of not wishing to tie up personal assets still exists for each of the investors.

Borrowing Money

Whether or not one personally has the necessary money, it usually will be advantageous to borrow most of the funds. Some sources of money available to the new private practitioner are investors, banks, and the Small Business Administration.

Investors

Investors are willing to loan money as a form of investment. They invest in the business instead of in a stock, bond, or mutual fund. They expect a fair return on their investment, which may be in the form of stock shares, interest on the money, or profit sharing. Innovative strategies can be devised to lure investors to the practice, but one must keep in mind the possibility that the investor may desire some control over the practice. If this is the situation, the sacrifice of control may be too great a price to pay for the initial funds.

Banks

Banks are a primary source of funding for new business; however, when investing they look for businesses that are sure to succeed. Small businesses have an inherently poor track record, many not surviving past the third year. This makes bankers nervous about making loans to small businesses.

When banks lend money to small businesses or to anyone, they are making judgments on the ability of the borrower to repay the loan. If the business appears vulnerable, banks may not wish to loan the funds, or if they are willing to do so, the terms of the loan may prove prohibitive to the new business. It should be remembered that new businesses look vulnerable essentially because they have no record of prior success. Accordingly, banks are more apt to loan money to those that are not in dire need than to those that are. Banks, like investors, are looking to benefit from the money they lend. They expect to receive income from the interest payments on the loan, and they hope to profit from providing banking services to the small business.

Small Business Administration

The Small Business Administration is a federal agency whose purpose is to help small businesses, to which it is empowered to make loans. It may loan funds directly up to $150,000 or, in participation with other lending agencies, up to a maximum of $500,000. To facilitate loans to small businesses, the Small Business Administration will guarantee up to 90 percent of the loan amount. Therefore, if the borrower defaults on the repayment, the lender loses at most only 10 percent of the loaned amount. This considerably reduces the risk to the lending institution.

Small Business Investment Companies

Small business investment companies represent another way in which the Small Business Administration can assist in financing small businesses. These privately owned investment companies are licensed and regulated by the federal government. They provide another means of the government trying to assist small businesses.

TYPES OF FUNDING

When money is borrowed, it may take the form of either cash, a credit line, or a conventional loan.

Cash

Cash is the type of money usually provided by the owner or owners of the business, who deposit their cash in the bank account of the private practice. Private investors may also provide cash to the business based upon the agreement of reimbursement to the investors.

Credit Line

A credit line is a form of loan in which the borrower is approved for a maximum amount of money from a lender. The borrower can borrow any or all of the approved amount for use in the business. However, there are usually stipulations attached to the credit line. A frequent stipulation is that for 30 days per year the credit line must have a zero loan balance. Another is that money spent to purchase capital equipment will be reclassified as a conventional loan.

The primary advantage of a credit line is that the borrower only pays interest on the money actually borrowed, not on the amount available for borrowing. If money is sought for short-term needs, this arrangement may prove most beneficial. However, to secure the credit line, the lending agency will require documentation that the borrowed money can be repaid. Therefore, this form of funding may prove best for a private practice that is already set up and functioning rather than one in the initial stages of formation.

Conventional Loans

When a loan is secured from a lender, it will have specific terms, including stipulations of the number of years, the type of interest, prepayment or balloon payments, and acquisition costs.

Duration of the Loan

One of the major considerations when securing a loan for a new private practice is the time during which the full amount of the loan must be repaid with interest. Banks usually do not wish to lend money beyond 3 years. They may allow 5 years for a loan used primarily for physical therapy equipment because if the practitioner defaults on the loan, the lender owns the equipment. However, physical therapy equipment is not what lending institutions wish to own. Also, the value of the equipment depreciates each year. The Small Business Administration is usually willing to grant a 7- to 10-year loan to the new private practice.

The duration of the loan is critical to the new private practice, as it directly affects the amount of the monthly payments to the lending institution. The following example illustrates the wide variation in monthly payments based upon a loan of $100,000 over loan periods of 1 to 9 years at a fixed 12 percent interest rate. The amount of the monthly payment includes the repayment of principal and interest.

$100,000 borrowed for	1 Year	3 Years	5 Years	7 Years	9 Years
Monthly Payment	$8,885	$3,321	$2,224	$1,765	$1,518

The above payments are made every month for the duration of the loan. By multiplying the monthly payment by the number of months one can calculate the total amount of money that has to be repaid on the borrowed amount.

Number of Payments	12	36	60	84	108
Total Repayment	$106,620	$119,556	$133,440	$148,260	$163,944

The above amounts of repayment clearly show why lending institutions are willing to loan money—they make a profit from the repayment schedule. For the private practitioner, selection of the number of years and the amount of each monthly payment represents critical decisions. A new private practitioner choosing the $100,000 loan for 1 year would have to make monthly payments of $8,885. A new business able to meet this payment schedule would be unique. On the other hand, the shorter the length of the loan, the less the total amount to be repaid. In the actual situation of a new private practitioner, the object is to obtain as much funding as needed and keep the monthly payment as low as possible. A long-term loan would most likely serve the new practitioner the best because in a new business the most difficult time is the early months, when cash flow is tight and it is hard to meet all the monthly obligations.

Rate of Interest

Equally as important as the duration of the loan are the type and rate of interest. The loan is usually of either a fixed-rate or variable-rate type. In a fixed-rate loan, the rate of interest remains constant for the length of the loan, as in the example used above of a $100,000 loan at a fixed 12 percent interest rate. With this fixed-rate loan the private practitioner knows that the monthly payment of principal and interest is the same every month that the loan is outstanding.

In a variable-rate loan the rate usually varies every month or every quarter, usually in relation to the prime interest rate (i.e., the rate at which banks borrow money). These loans are generally a few percentage points above the prime interest rate. The following example is presented to show how the difference in interest rate will affect the monthly expense for a 7-year loan of $100,000.

Interest rate (%)	9	10	11	12	13	14	15	16
Monthly payment	$1,609	$1,660	$1,712	$1,765	$1,819	$1,874	$1,930	$1,986

In this example, the difference from one percentage point to the next is approximately $50. In the case of a fixed-rate loan, this means $50 more that the practitioner pays to the lender every month for each percentage increase in rate; it amounts to $600.00 per year and $4,200.00 over the 7-year life of the loan.

In the case of a variable-rate loan, the rate can vary from month to month or from quarter to quarter; it can rise and cost the practitioner more, or it can fall and cost the practitioner less. Therefore, the variable rate has some excitement attached to it, but the variation can be traumatic if the interest rate climbs abruptly and the practice is not in a financial position to handle the increased monthly cost.

Schedule of Payments

In securing a loan one question that needs to be addressed is the ability to repay the loan early. Some loans have a *prepayment penalty,* which the borrower pays if the loan is repaid faster than agreed upon. This penalty is usually spelled out when the loan is made. Some loans allow advance payment of a portion of the loan each year, and any such additional payment incurs a penalty. The purpose of such a stipulation is to allow the lending institution to earn the revenue it expects from the loan. When a loan is paid, the payment is broken down into *principal,* which is the portion of the loan payment that is used to offset the money borrowed, and *interest* the amount of money paid to the lender as the fee for the use of the lender's money.

Some loans permit repayment in advance. The right to do this is called *no prepayment penalty*. Private practitioners, when their cash flow problems diminish, have to decide if prepayment is in their best interest. If the practitioner prepays, then the amount of the loan decreases, and either the monthly payments or the number of months remaining on the loan decrease. This facilitates the private practitioner's chances of borrowing future funds. However, the loan prepayment serves as an expense to the business, and the business's accountant may feel that not prepaying the loan may better serve the practice from a tax viewpoint.

Another type of loan payback schedule is called a *balloon*. In this arrangement the initial payments are relatively low to help the new practitioner make ends meet. At some predetermined time the loan must be paid in full or the payments increase to a higher level. This works well providing that the practitioner is prepared to make larger payments or the full repayment. At times this type of loan is essential, as a new business may need to start with the smallest possible monthly repayment schedule.

Loan Acquisition Costs

One more item to consider when trying to secure financing is acquisition costs, which are the costs associated with securing the loan. These may include payment to a person who helps prepare the formal documents for the loan and the attorney fee for the closing. Fees paid to the city, state, or federal government would be considered in this category. Loan officers are able to provide an estimate of the loan acquisition costs, which are usually expressed in terms of *points*. These points are synonymous with percentage points; thus, a two-point acquisition cost on a $100,000 loan equals $2,000. This cost is paid by the borrower when closing the loan or is subtracted from the cash received from the loan.

STEPS IN SECURING FINANCING

To be willing to lend money to a new business, a lender must believe that the owners of the new venture have a strong chance to succeed or if not succeed, at least repay the loan. Therefore, most lending institutions have developed criteria for evaluating prospective new businesspeople and new ventures. Some of the criteria frequently evaluated by lenders are (1) the ability of the borrowers to repay the loan; and (2) the potential for the new business to succeed.

Ability of Borrowers to Repay Loan

To assess ability to repay the loan, lending institutions request personal financial statements from all the borrowers for a proposed new venture. A personal financial statement gives an up-to-date picture of the financial solvency of the borrower. It is usually divided into sections labeled *Assets* and *Liabilities,* and includes information concerning sources and amounts of the borrower's income and expenses (Fig. 3-1).

The lending institution supplies the potential borrower with a form to complete, which requests the necessary information, including account numbers, addresses, and any other data that facilitate checking the accuracy of the information supplied. The more precise the potential borrower is in presenting the necessary information, the more quickly the lending institution can process the application.

In the section entitled Assets the following information is usually requested:

1. *Cash on hand or in the bank:* The amount of money easily accessible, including cash, savings accounts, checking accounts, and money market funds
2. *Retirement accounts or annuities:* The cash value of accounts not considered easily accessible
3. *Accounts receivable:* Money owed to and expected to be received by the potential borrower
4. *Life insurance (cash surrender value):* The value of life insurance policies if cashed in during the life of the insured
5. *Stocks and bonds:* The current value of presently owned stocks and bonds
6. *Real estate:* The current value of presently owned real estate
7. *Automobiles:* The current value of presently owned automobiles
8. *Personal property:* The present value of personal items owned
9. *Other assets:* All presently owned assets not listed above

Upon completing each of these nine items, the potential borrower adds the amounts listed and enters the sum on the line entitled Total Assets.

A similar procedure is followed for the section entitled Liabilities, which identifies to the lending institution how much money the borrower owes and to whom. The information requested is as follows:

1. *Accounts payable:* Money the potential borrower owes to others
2. *Notes payable:* Currently outstanding notes or loans that are being paid in some fashion, usually monthly (including automobile or school loans, which should be listed separately)
3. *Loans against life insurance:* Money already borrowed against life insurance policies (which reduces the face value of the life insurance if not repaid)
4. *Mortgages on real estate:* The total amount of money owed on real estate owned by the borrower
5. *Unpaid taxes:* Taxes owed by the borrower
6. *Other liabilities:* Any unpaid debts not listed above that the borrower has incurred

Upon completing these six items, the potential borrower adds the amounts listed and enters the sum in the line entitled Total Liabilities.

The cumulative liabilities are now subtracted from the cumulative assets, and the difference is entered on the line entitled Net Worth. Obviously, if the potential

Personal Financial Statement

Name: _____

Address: _____

Assets	**Liabilities**
Cash	Accounts Payable
Retirement Accounts and Annuities	Notes Payable
Accounts Receivable	Loans Against Life Insurance
Life Insurance (Cash Surrender Value)	Mortgages on Real Estate
Stocks and Bonds	Unpaid Taxes
Real Estate	Other Liabilities
Automobiles	
Personal Property	
Other	

Total Assets _____   Total Liabilities _____

    Total Assets

– Total Liabilities

    _____

    Net Worth

Sources of Income

Salary

Net Investment Income

Real Estate Income

Other Income

Total Income _____

Fig. 3-1. Personal financial statement.

borrower has low assets or high liabilities, the lending institution will not be pleased with the personal profile presented.

The personal financial statement contains an additional section concerning sources of income, which informs the lending institution about how large the potential borrower's income is and from what sources it is derived. The same procedure is used for completing this section as was used for the assets and liabilities sections. The information requested is

1. *Salary:* Salary from present avenues of employment
2. *Net investment income:* Income from present investments, such as stocks and bonds
3. *Real estate income:* Income from owned real estate, such as rental income
4. *Other income:* Income not listed above (e.g., alimony or child support)

Upon completing this section, the potential borrower adds the amounts listed for each item and enters the sum on the line entitled Total Income.

The sections on assets, liabilities, and income cover the primary information requested by lending institutions from prospective borrowers. Specific lending institutions may use their own forms and ask for additional information.

In addition to the personal financial statement, most lending institutions will request that the potential borrower submit tax returns from the last year or the last 2 years. This allows the lending institution to assess the stability of the prospective borrower's financial situation.

It is conceivable that a lending institution will refuse to loan funds to a new business. This is especially true because the rate of failure of new businesses is high. Therefore it is imperative that the persons borrowing the money on behalf of the private practice be capable of repaying the loan. Most lending institutions will require personal guarantees when lending funds to new businesses. These are documents signed by the individual borrowers stating that they individually accept responsibility for the loaned amount. The lender is thereby protected in the event that the private practice does not succeed, as the individual borrowers would still be responsible for paying off the loan.

Once the lending institution has been assured that the borrowers of the funds will be able to repay the loan if the new venture does not succeed, it must assess the new business's chance to become successful.

Potential for the New Business to Succeed

When applying for a business loan, the applicant must provide a sufficient amount of information about the business to the potential lender. Some of the items that must be included are

1. Information about the organization
2. Information about the owners
3. Location of facility
4. Amount of money requested
5. Start-up costs

6. Equipment and supply purchases
7. Monthly operating expenses
8. How the loan proceeds will be used
9. Revenue projections

Information about the Organization

In a short written statement the potential private practitioners should explain to the lender what the organization is all about. This statement should give the name of the private practice, its legal format (sole proprietorship, partnership, or corporation), and the names of the owners and investors. If the structure of the organization has some unique features, these should be explained. Any special situation that demonstrates the organization's potential ability to repay the loan must be described. One such situation occurs when there are multiple owners, some of whom maintain their employment in outside organizations. This ensures salary income and demonstrates that the new practice intends to not drain its finances, as the owners with outside employment may not require an up-front salary from the new business.

Included in this statement must be an explanation of how the private practice expects to succeed. This discussion may need to be prefaced by an explanation of what physical therapy and physical therapists are. It should highlight market research by the owners or companies hired by the owners that shows a community need for the practice. For example, market research may show that there are only a few physical therapy practices in the chosen community, that there are only a few hospitals providing outpatient physical therapy, and that the local physical therapy facilities all have waiting lists for patients in need of such treatment. As a second example, market research may show that the physical therapy available in a community is geared to meet only the needs of patients with a specific type of problem. If the new practice is geared to the needs of patients who are being placed on waiting lists or not being served, this would be viewed as a positive factor by the potential lending institution.

Accordingly, showing the potential lender that the practitioners have investigated the new community and have a viable plan will enhance the chances for approval of the loan application. The negative alternative is to apply for a loan with no real organized plan for the success of the practice.

Information about the Owners

The easiest way to present information to the potential lending institution about the owners is by including curricula vitae or resumes for each of the owners, which present organized and chronologically ordered career histories. In addition to these career histories, anything unique about one or more of the owners must be called to the potential lender's attention, for example, if one or more owners have successfully started and built up a private practice in another location. Such a record of success, which can be documented with financial information from the previous practice, clearly enhances the chances for approval of the new private practice's loan application.

Location of the Facility

Investigation of the community and careful selection of an office location show the potential lender that the new practice will be headed by serious and thoughtful practitioners. The fact that the organization has moved forward by selecting the location makes a favorable impression. The owners could present a copy of the lease or the proposed lease with the loan application. Once again, this signifies the advanced stage of development of the new private practice and will strongly impress lending institutions.

Amount Requested

When it comes to requesting funds for the new practice, the owners must decide how much funding is necessary, how much is adequate, and how much represents luxury. The *necessary* amount of money is the minimal amount needed by the new venture to have a chance of succeeding. The *adequate* amount is the amount that it must have to launch the practice with minimal hardship to the owners. The *luxury* amount is the amount that would provide the practice with all possible luxuries.

When money is borrowed, the lender does not want to assume all the risk. One common way to share the risk is for the owners to invest some of their own money in the venture. When a lending institution limits the amount of money it is willing to lend to the new practice, the practitioners must either alter their plans or increase their personal investment. This situation affects the developmental plan of the business. Adequate funding implies that the lending institution and the owners have enough funds between them to develop a sound practice with a good chance of success. A minimal funding situation occurs when funds available from the lending institution and the owners together are insufficient and the business plan has to be revised downward to accommodate the fiscal reality.

When presenting the financial needs of a new venture to a lending institution, the costs must be carefully spelled out, usually by preparing statements of start-up costs, equipment and supply purchases, and monthly operating expenses.

Start-up Costs

There are many start-ups costs for a new business, which may present a problem because the new entrepreneur usually is not aware of some of them until after they have materialized. This may lead to inadequate projection of total start-up costs, in which case operating dollars will have to be used to pay for some of them. This puts the new business at a disadvantage before its doors have ever opened.

Start-up costs are one-time expenses that occur prior to the opening of the practice. If these costs reoccur, they are considered part of the operating expenses, but when the new practice has yet to open, the initial expenses obviously cannot be so considered. Additionally, start-up costs can be rather large and must be anticipated so that funds can be made available to pay these early bills.

Some of the start-up costs are presented below.

Legal Fees

The owners will incur fees for the services of an attorney in developing the necessary legal documents. These include the articles of incorporation, shareholder agreements, and employee contracts. Additional tasks of the attorney are to file the appropriate papers with the state if a corporation is set up and to provide legal advice when indicated. Additionally, the attorney must read and try to improve any rental agreement between the private practice and the landlord (see Ch. 4).

Rental Deposits

A deposit is normally paid to the landlord, usually in the amount of one month's rent. Another form of rental deposit would be money forwarded to the landlord or to a contractor for office renovations that have been agreed upon by the owners of the practice and the landlord before occupation of the leased space.

Office Buildout or Enhancements

Additional expenses are costs of specific structural work to the office before occupancy, this may include plumbing, walls, electrical outlets, and special flooring. These items are negotiable between the potential lessee (the private practitioner) and the lessor (the landlord). Remember that the landlord will always strive to pass on as much of the expense as possible to the new private practitioner. Through negotiations the landlord can generally be induced to incur some of the costs.

Prepaid Rent

Prepayments of rent to the landlord may be made for an arbitrary number of months, usually the first and last months of the lease. However, it is usually possible through negotiation for the new private practitioner to arrange to occupy the premises rent-free for a variable number of months.

Office Supplies

Printed materials are necessary for running the practice and letting other people know that the practice exists. Some of the needed items are business cards, letterhead stationery, envelopes, referral pads, and billing forms. It is not uncommon to pay a graphic designer to design a logo for the new private practice. Some of the other office supplies required for efficient functioning of the private practice include file folders, pens and pencils, paper, and paper clips.

Advertising

Expenses are incurred to promote the new business before and during the life of the practice. Those advertising expenses incurred before opening are considered start-up costs. Advertisements in telephone directories and announcements of the grand opening in newspapers fit into this category.

Utility Deposits

Utility deposits are payments, analogous to rental deposits, that are made to the local electric, water, and telephone companies. Since the new business does not have a credit record, these companies usually request deposits before initiating service.

Other Start-Up Expenses

License fees are expenses associated with obtaining licenses to open the business. These are not the physical therapy licenses, which also require a fee, but permits from the city, county, and state to operate a business within their respective jurisdictions.

Insurance premiums must be paid before validation of the respective insurance policies. Some forms of insurance are malpractice, office liability, and medical.

Educational expenses incurred before opening the practice are considered start-up costs. Such expenses may cover continuing education for the owners or the staff, library reference texts, or business management consultant services.

Architectural fees are usually paid to an architect for helping to design the new office to specifications.

Accountant fees are paid to an accountant to develop an accounting system for the new practice.

Estimation of Total Start-up Costs

The above discussion includes many of the start-up costs that new private practitioners will incur. It is impossible to present here even a "ball park" dollar estimate for these costs. To assess accurately the magnitude of these costs, a future private practitioner should investigate many of these items through telephone calls and personal meetings with the many service providers. Another method of assessing these costs is to speak with established private practitioners in the state and community and try to get a feel for these expenses. The more vigorously these inquires are pursued, the more accurate will be the practitioner's estimate for the start-up costs. Moreover, operating dollars will not be needed to compensate for a poor estimate of start-up costs. It should be realized that these expenses are one-time expenses that can be of considerable magnitude.

Equipment and Supply Purchases

When developing the philosophy of the new practice the owners should also develop a list of necessary equipment. Certain basic equipment is needed for most physical therapy practices. In addition, various specialized equipment

Table 3-1. Physical Therapy Equipment and Supplies

Basic equipment
- Hydrocollator unit
- Cold pack unit
- Treatment plinths
- Traction unit
- Paraffin bath
- Ultrasound unit
- Electrical stimulation unit
- Whirlpool unit
- Whirlpool chair
- Free and cuff weights
- Sphygmomanometer
- Stethoscope
- Chairs
- Canes
- Crutches
- Walkers

Variable equipment
- Isotonic weight machines
- Isokinetic machine
- Electric Hi-Lo treatment plinths
- Stationary bicycles
- Treadmills
- Biofeedback machine
- Wheelchairs

Supplies
- Hot packs
- Hot pack covers
- Ice packs
- Towels
- Ultrasound gel
- Massage lotion
- Traction accessories
- Paraffin
- Quad board
- Theraband
- Lumbar corsets

- Lumbar rolls
- Patient educational aids
- Linen

Office equipment
- Telephones
- Telephone answering machine
- Calculator or adding machine
- Typewriter
- Copying machine
- Filing cabinet

Furniture
- Office chairs
- Desks
- Waiting room chairs
- Waiting room couches
- Waiting room tables
- Lamps

Computer hardware and software
- Computer
- Keyboard
- Monitor
- Printer
- Software package

Pantry items
- Refrigerator
- Microwave oven
- Coffee machine
- Water cooler
- Clothes washer
- Clothes dryer

Fixtures
- Pictures
- Mirrors
- Carpeting
- Special lighting

would be required for those clinics with specific goals. An example of a specialized need is isokinetic equipment for a practice that expects a large influx of orthopedic patients. With this in mind, equipment needs may be broken down into basic and specialized. Physical therapy supplies must be considered. Other categories of purchases may include office equipment, office furniture, computer hardware and software, pantry equipment, and office fixtures. A listing of many of these items can be found in Table 3-1.

The items to be purchased are either required for or desired by physical therapy practices. When applying for initial funding it is advantageous to separate the items desired so that the loan officer can tell what the equipment portion of the loan is going to fund. The amount and cost of equipment desired for the new private practice will directly affect the start-up cost. The more expensive and the greater the amount of the equipment purchased, the larger will be the initial funding required. A method to decrease the dollar amount required to purchase equipment items would be to lease some items for a monthly fee. The lease is an agreement made with the company that sells the equipment or with a leasing company that buys the equipment from the manufacturer and then leases it to the private practice. A lease of equipment is nothing more than an agreement to pay a monthly fee for its use. Usually, at the end of the agreed-upon number of months or years of the lease, the user has the right to buy the equipment for a predetermined fee. The benefit of this to the private practice is that it reduces the amount of up-front money necessary to start the practice; however, it increases monthly operating expenses. Additionally, at the end of the lease the private practice will have paid more for the leased equipment over the length of the lease than if the equipment had been bought outright when the practice was started.

Monthly Operating Expenses

When starting a new business venture it is important in the initial funding to include monies for monthly operating costs. Funding for 12 months of operation would be luxurious although not realistic. Six months of operating funds should be sufficient. The money for monthly operations is imperative as collections inevitably lag behind the dates of treatment rendered and treatment billed (see Ch. 12).

Once again, determining the actual operating expenses is based on knowledge already gained and calculated guesses. The primary monthly expenses for operating a physical therapy practice are discussed below.

Salaries

Salaries are the monthly amounts paid to the employees of the organization, including physical therapists, administrators, secretaries, and any other employees who receive regular paychecks. For convenience of the loan application this item may be reported as the yearly salary of all employees divided by 12 months. As the practice grows more employees may be added, but for the purpose of obtaining the loan it is not usually necessary to project cost estimates into the distant future.

Payroll Taxes

Payroll taxes are the amounts of federal income tax withheld by management when paying employees their salaries. The cumulative total of payroll taxes withheld by the business is transferred to the bank monthly for submission to the federal and, in some states, the state government. Payroll taxes do not cost the business additional money as they are included in the salary item. However, it may benefit the owners of the practice to know what the net pay on a gross salary will be, since many new private practitioners accept a lesser salary.

Social Security Withholdings

The amount of money withheld by the private practice from employee salaries for payment into the U.S. Social Security system is, like the payroll taxes, deposited monthly with the bank, in this case for submission to the Social Security Administration. The private practice has to match the dollar amount of employee contributions; thus, Social Security contributions represent a cost to the private practice. Additionally, if the owner(s) of this practice are on salary, they must pay twice for the employee contribution, both as a paycheck deduction and as the matching share from the business. The cost of the employee contribution changes, usually yearly. As of 1988, the cost of the employee contribution was 7.51 percent of the gross paycheck up to $48,000. Social Security employee contributions do not cost the private practice additional funds as they are included in the salary item, but the matching share contribution does cost the owners additional money. This amount can be calculated in advance and included in the loan application.

Additional Taxes

Every quarter, following the accountant's review of the appropriate information, some minor additional taxes may be due. The amount of these should be minimal and cannot be predicted in advance by a new practice.

Rent

Rent is the amount the private practice agrees to pay the landlord for the use of the office. This amount is usually fixed for a period of time, most often one year, but when a lease is negotiated, the rent may be frozen for a longer period. The change in rent is usually tied to the consumer price index, which is the monthly cost of living index for the average person.

Frequently, there is an annual additional expense for building-related costs that exceed the landlord's budget projection. This expense is usually distributed to all the tenants based on square footage rented.

Loan Repayment

The practitioners agree to pay the financial lender a specified amount for use of the borrowed funds. After deciding on start-up costs, equipment and supply purchases, and monthly operating expenses, the owners are able to determine the financial needs of the practice, which guides them in determining the amount to be requested from the lending institution. From their best estimates of the above items the practitioners are able to calculate the amount of the monthly loan repayment. Obviously, the owners have to make assumptions regarding the length and interest rate of the loan. However, the fact that they present a calculation of the repayment amount should favorably impress the lending institution, as it shows good business sense.

Utility Expenses

Utility costs to be considered are those for electricity, water, and telephone services. The electricity and water costs may already be included in the monthly rent; however, if this is not the case, the practitioners will have to guess the monthly costs of these services. By communicating with other private practitioners in the area and adapting their cost data to the physical size and unique electrical needs of the new office they can obtain an initial estimate.

Telephone service can be partially estimated from information supplied by the telephone company. The monthly service charge is determined by the number of telephones and the number of telephone lines to the office. Additionally, the cost of advertising in the telephone book is usually paid on a monthly basis. The primary variable is the use of long-distance services, since charges vary considerably among long-distance carriers. Obviously, the amount of long-distance telephone calls will affect the monthly cost of this service.

Office Cleaning

The cost of maintaining the office in a clean and orderly condition may be included in the rent. However, if this is not the case, the new practitioner will have to pay for a cleaning service.

Medical Supplies

The monthly costs of medical supplies, which are items needed for the actual provision of physical therapy services (ultrasound gel, rubber gloves, electrodes, etc.), must be estimated. Communication with other private practitioners may be the best way to estimate this cost.

Office Supplies

The monthly cost of supplies needed for the efficient running of the office (typewriter ribbons, paper, rubber bands, postage, etc.) must be estimated. Here, also, communication with other private practitioners may lead to the best estimation.

Continuing Education

Money allocated for educating the staff of the new practice is usually considered an annual expense. For the purpose of allocating funds the annual amount is divided by 12 so that monthly amounts can be budgeted.

Accounting and Legal Expenses

Monthly costs will be incurred for the services of the private practice's accountant and attorney. The accountant has many responsibilities to the new practice during the year (see Ch. 4). The lawyer, however, does not have many responsibilities to the practice after the initial documents have been completed and the contracts negotiated and signed (see Ch. 4). Therefore, the accountant will cost more than the lawyer. The annual expenses for each can be estimated on the basis of discussions with the accountant and the attorney and then divided by 12 to obtain the corresponding monthly amounts.

Insurance Premiums

Premiums are the amounts to keep insurance policies in force. Insurance policies for a private physical therapy practice may include malpractice, office liability, and health insurance. If these premiums are paid annually or quarterly, they can be prorated on a monthly basis.

Dues and Subscriptions

Additional costs are those for membership in physical therapy organizations and for purchase of magazines for the library and waiting room. Membership costs can be fixed from the outset, and a specific amount can be allocated for subscriptions. These costs can be calculated on a monthly basis.

Public Relations

Costs related to marketing the new business are considered public relations expenses. The success of the business will be directly related to how well known it becomes (see Ch. 11). Since this is critical for the success of the practice, the owners may wish to consider allocating a large amount of money to this item. However, many public relations items do not cost much. Therefore, the owners must decide on their marketing strategy and allocate an appropriate annual amount, which can be divided by 12 to obtain a monthly figure, although the expenses may not be incurred each month.

Miscellaneous Expenses

It may prove beneficial to allocate 10 percent of the expected monthly expenditure to miscellaneous items that have not been considered in advance.

Summary of Monthly Operating Expenses

The above discussion is presented to make the new private practitioners aware of the many expenses involved. In their efforts to secure funding for the new venture, they should realize that the lending institution is interested in knowing how much money will be needed to pay monthly bills. The lending institution will consider the start-up costs and the monthly operating costs in relation to revenue projections before deciding to approve a loan.

Use of the Loan Proceeds

When a lending institution evaluates a loan application, it prefers to grant funds for tangible expenditures, such as purchase of equipment. In this case the lending institution takes a lien on the equipment, of which it will acquire ownership in the event that the borrower defaults on the loan. This provides the

Table 3-2. Start-up Costs

Item	Cost
Legal fees	0,000
Rental deposits	0,000
Office buildout	0,000
Prepaid rent	0,000
Office supplies	0,000
Advertising	0,000
Utility deposits	0,000
License fees	0,000
Insurance premiums	0,000
Education expenses	0,000
Architectural fees	0,000
Accountant fees	0,000
Total	00,000

lending institution with a tangible asset as a form of collateral. Money borrowed for working capital provides no tangible asset and therefore is less desirable. Since most lending institutions require the owners of the new practice to invest some of their own money, the owners' investment is specified for use as the working capital, and the loan proceeds are specified for equipment purchases, office renovations, and start-up costs. To clearly inform the lending institutions, the three areas of financial need—start-up costs, equipment purchases, and monthly operating expenses—are commonly spelled out in chart form, usually as appendixes to the loan application (Tables 3-2 to 3-4).

When requesting financial assistance for the new private practice, money for start-up costs and equipment is not enough; money must be provided at the start to cover operating expenses for the first six months. The lack of funds to meet cash flow needs is one of the biggest reasons for failure among new businesses. In view of the fact that insurance reimbursement may take 30 to 90 days after billing for services rendered, the minimum cash needed for operating expenses has to be enough for 6 months. It is far better to have too much than too little operating cash.

Table 3-3. Equipment Purchases

Quantity	Manufacturer	Catalog No.	Description/Model	Cost	Cost Subtotal[a]
1	Y	111	Hydrocollator	0,000	0,000
1	Y	222	Cold pack	0,000	0,000
4	P	333	Plinth	0,000	0,000
1	Q	444	Traction	0,000	0,000
...	...	...	...	...	...
	Total				00,000

[a] All equipment purchases are to be listed with the above information and the cost subtotals added to give the grand total.

Table 3-4. Monthly Operating Expenses

Item	Cost
Salaries	
Owner 1	0,000
Staff therapist 1	0,000
Staff therapist 2	0,000
Secretary	0,000
Payroll taxes	0,000
Social Security	0,000
Additional taxes	0,000
Rent	0,000
Loan	0,000
Utilities	0,000
Office cleaning	0,000
Medical supplies	0,000
Office supplies	0,000
Continuing education	0,000
Accounting/legal fees	0,000
Insurance	0,000
Dues and subscriptions	0,000
Public relations	0,000
Miscellaneous	0,000
Total	00,000

Revenue Projections

Once the new private practitioner has explained to the lending institution how the loan proceeds are to be used, it is imperative to show the institution how the practice will be able to generate sufficient revenue to repay the loan and pay all the other bills.

For the purpose of discussion, assume that the new private physical therapy practice has one owner, paid on salary, who serves as both the administrator and the staff physical therapist. Monthly operating expenses have been calculated as $10,000. The lending institution must be shown that the practice can generate $10,000 per month to pay all bills and has the potential for making a profit to cover rising costs.

Physical therapists know that referred patients usually receive physical therapy two or three times per week. Therefore each physical therapy referral may be considered to be worth 2½ physical therapy treatments per week. One must make an educated guess as to the actual reimbursement for the treatments, as this will vary from one geographic location to another and will also vary depending on the patient population treated. Medicare, Workers' Compensation, health maintenance organization, and private pay patients all generate different dollar amounts per treatment session. As a result of the new practice's research, an estimated dollar figure should be assumed. For example, $40.00 can be anticipated as the reimbursement for each therapy session. This figure would take into account high payers (over $40.00) and low payers (under $40.00). If one wishes to consider the gross billings and subtract the bad debts (i.e., money not

Table 3-5. Weekly Income

Week No.	No. of Patients	No. of Treatments	Income ($)
1	1	2.5	100
2	3	7.5	300
3	5	12.5	500
4	7	17.5	700
	First month income		1,600
5	9	22.5	900
6	11	27.5	1,100
7	13	32.5	1,300
8	15	37.5	1,500
	Second month income		4,800
9	17	42.5	1,700
10	19	47.5	1,900
11	21	52.5	2,100
12	23	57.5	2,300
	Third month income		8,000
13	25	62.5	2,500
14	27	67.5	2,700
15	29	72.5	2,900
16	31	77.5	3,100
	Fourth month income		11,200
17	33	82.5	3,300
18	35	87.5	3,500
19	37	92.5	3,700
20	39	97.5	3,900
	Fifth month income		14,400

collected from the billings), the reimbursement could be estimated on the basis of $50.00 billed per treatment and 20 percent bad debts, for a net collection of $40.00 per treatment. Remember that these figures are arbitrarily assumed at the time of the loan application. When the practice has been operating for about 6 months, the owner can determine the actual rate of reimbursement per treatment. Additionally, instead of the reimbursement per treatment, the reimbursement per procedure (e.g., hot pack, therapeutic exercise, electrical stimulation) may be used. This creates more variables and therefore makes the preparation of the loan documents more cumbersome.

The following example is based on the assumption that each referral results in 2½ visits per week at $40.00 per visit and that the practice is growing by two new referrals per week. On speaking with other private practitioners, it will become apparent to the new private therapist that this is a slow rate of growth. Even with this conservative projection, the potential for the new practice will be shown to be sound. Remember that the monthly operating expenses for this example are assumed to amount to $10,000. A likely pattern of income growth during the first several months of operation is shown in Table 3-5.

On the basis of these projections it will take approximately 4 months for the new private practice to generate enough business to break even. Additionally at this point reimbursement should start to be received for the patients treated during the earlier months, so the amount of cash received should be close to that of the bills generated. The slow growth rate of only two new patients per week does allow for discharge of patients. The type of patient referred will affect the length of therapy services. For example, a neurologic patient or one with an anterior cruciate ligament repair would require more therapy than one with a mild ankle sprain.

At this point the prospective private practitioner may be thinking that setting up a practice appears too easy—there must be a "catch." There *is* a catch. As the business grows, business expenses grow. At some point in the above situation the visits will exceed the capabilities of one therapist. Therefore a second therapist must be hired, and a second office person may also be needed. More patients visits may require more supplies, greater mailing costs, etc. To account for these extra costs, for the fifth month a $4,000 increase in expenses may be assumed. Now the monthly operating expenses are $14,000. The projections for the fifth month are shown in Table 3-5.

After 5 months the practice is again at the break-even point, but this time the new therapists may have picked up approximately 20 additional visits as compared with the last month. Now the practice can generate a profit on the additional 40 or more visits the second therapist will produce before a third therapist is required. Variations in personnel costs, such as those of hiring physical therapy assistants or aides, will result in variations in income generated and expenses. Lending institutions usually wish to see this kind of revenue and expenditure projection for the first year. This can be charted on a monthly basis in whatever fashion the lending institution desires.

SUMMARY

This chapter discusses how to apply for initial funding to start a private physical therapy practice. The steps involved consist of deciding on where to apply for funding, the type of funding needed, the loan amount and terms, and the steps required to secure funding.

SUGGESTED READINGS

Circular E. Employer's Tax Guide. Internal Revenue Service, Florence, KY, 1989

Deaton C: Your Private Practice—Financial Planning. Ben E. Johnston Jr. & Peter J. Lord, Lake City, FL, 1982

Greene GG: How to Start and Manage Your Own Business, 3rd Ed. New American Library, New York, 1983

J.K. Lasser Tax Institute: How to Run a Small Business. 6th Ed. McGraw-Hill, New York, 1983

Krentzman HC: Successful Management Strategies for Small Business. Prentice-Hall, Englewood Cliffs, NJ, 1981

Mancuso JR: How to Prepare and Present a Business Plan. Prentice-Hall Press, New York, 1983

The Complete Payment Book. Contemporary Books, Chicago, 1983

Talamo J: The Real Estate Dictionary. 4th Ed. Financial Publishing Co., Boston, 1986

4

SUPPORT SYSTEMS

Development of a successful private practice requires considerable support from other professionals. To receive the necessary support and subsequent counseling every private practice must develop and cultivate its own support systems. Private practitioners should call on their support systems at the right time.

ATTORNEY

An attorney is essential to the developing physical therapy practice. The legal counsel selected should serve four primary purposes: conceptual advice, legal documentation, employment agreements, and negotiations. The corporate structure will be assumed in the following discussion of the functions of the attorney.

Conceptual Advice

During the conceptual stage of a private practice the potential owner(s) envision what the practice will be like. Most physical therapists can visualize the practice but do not understand the legal implications. Therefore, at the first meeting with the selected attorney the physical therapist should present the format of the planned private practice. The lawyer, after listening to the physical therapist's description of the new business, may recommend various alternative legal structures. This discussion should make the physical therapist better equipped to select the formal structure for the private practice.

Legal Documentation

Once the legal structure is chosen, the lawyer must then file the appropriate documentation with the state. Some of these legal entities are as follows.

Corporate Name

After thorough consideration the owner(s) of the new physical therapy practice select a name for the practice. Providing that the corporate name chosen is available, the attorney secures this name legally for the practice.

Articles of Incorporation

The articles of incorporation is a document that must be filed with the appropriate state agency. This document states the name of the corporation, the corporation's purpose, and the number of shareholders. To become shareholders, the practitioners/investors of the private practice buy shares of stock. The document also lists the name and address of the private practice's registered agent, usually one of the practice's owners. After the corporation is formed, corporate by-laws are adopted. The by-laws describe the procedures under which the corporation functions.

Shareholders' Agreement

In conjunction with the articles of incorporation and the by-laws, the shareholders' agreement, when used, provides guidelines for the stockholders. The terms of the agreement represent the views of the shareholders. The attorney assists in conceptualizing the terms of the agreement and drafting it in the appropriate format.

The shareholders' agreement documents the names of the shareholders and the number of shares owned by each. Included in the document are the voting process, the requirements for meetings, and the actions allowed without meetings. A restrictive covenant among the shareholders may be included. A restrictive covenant restricts shareholders from competing with the corporation in a manner prohibited by the agreement. An example would be restricting one shareholder from opening a second physical therapy practice in the same neighborhood. Restrictive covenants must be reasonable. (See discussion on restrictive covenants under the employee agreement below.) This agreement may include requirements about the board of directors and shareholders who serve the practice as employees. The powers of the corporate officers should be included.

The shareholders' agreement should also discuss the rules and regulations concerning the sale or transfer of shares of stock and the process to be implemented if one of the shareholders should die. Also, it may prove helpful to describe a system of valuing shares of stock, which is done at the annual shareholders meeting. This agreement should also provide guidelines for handling any disagreement that may arise among shareholders.

Buy-Sell Agreement

The buy-sell agreement is an agreement among the shareholders about how shares of stock may be transferred or sold. Shareholders may wish to buy the shares of another shareholder or wish to sell their own shares of stock in the corporation. A buy-sell agreement providing guidelines for these situations can help prevent confusion. Changes in the body of shareholders may result from many causes, such as a shareholder's move to another part of the country or an unresolvable philosophical difference between two shareholders.

Many problems are inherent in buying and selling shares of the corporation. One problem is the dollar value placed on the shares. The selling shareholder wishes the value to be set high and the buying shareholder understandably wishes the value to be very low. Another problem may stem from the remaining shareholders perhaps not wanting outside parties to become shareholders. A clearly written and easy to enact buy-sell agreement can prevent many shareholder problems and their associated ill will.

Frequently, many new private physical therapy practices open without a buy-sell agreement. This initially saves money on legal fees and is not considered important, as the new corporation really has no significant dollar value. However, once the corporation becomes successful, it may prove very difficult to develop a buy-sell agreement among shareholders because people change and their philosophies change, especially in their views of a successful private practice.

Ordering Corporate Seal and Minute Book

The attorney normally orders the official corporate seal for the new corporation. The seal is used on official documents signed on behalf of the corporation, for example, when formally closing on loan documents. Corporations must maintain minutes of their annual and other meetings. The minutes can be maintained in the minute book. The attorney may write up the minutes of the initial meetings and start the book.

Issue Stock

Stock certificates are issued to each shareholder. The attorney frequently holds the stock certificates on behalf of the corporate stockholders.

Corporate Annual Maintenance

For a corporation to maintain good standing in the state in which it is incorporated it must follow the requirements of that state. Frequently a corporation, for a retainer fee, elects to assign this responsibility to its attorney. The attorney may hold the minute book and include in it the minutes of the corporation's annual meeting. The attorney may hold the certificates of stock. In addition, the attorney will insure that the corporation is up to date in complying with all state administrative requirements.

Employment Agreements

Employment agreements are formally drafted contracts between employer and employee. The employer is the private practice. The employee may be anyone hired by the practice. Agreements are more frequently executed with the professional than with the administrative staff.

Terms of Employment

Employment agreements state the terms of employment for the employee, which may include:

1. Length of employment and renewal options
2. Number of days notice required for termination of employment by either party
3. Employee responsibilities
4. Annual salary or other forms of compensation for services performed
5. Pay increase stipulations mutually agreed upon by employer and employee
6. Benefit package provided to the employee (vacation, holiday and sick leave policies, continuing education, medical benefits, liability coverage, etc.)

Reasons for termination of the employment need to be clearly spelled out to prevent potential conflicts, and responsibilities of both employer and employee upon termination must be outlined. One employer responsibility usually is that the employee must be paid the wages earned. A responsibility on the part of the employee is not to solicit business away from the employer (restrictive covenant).

Restrictive Covenants

The restrictive covenant, if part of the employment agreement, must be spelled out clearly. The purpose of the covenant is to protect the employer from losing business to the employee, a risk in every private business setting. The employer opens the door to the employees and provides a unique working environment. Through knowledge, gained by working for the employer, the employees acquire the potential to leave and open their own physical therapy facility. If the employees compete with the employer, they most likely will use information learned through their employment. With a restrictive covenant, the employer is able to deal with employees openly without fear of potential harm to the practice.

The following hypothetical situation may well follow if no restrictive covenant is in place. During employment in a private practice, an employee provides patient care for two specific referring physicians. The employee, after developing a strong professional relationship with these physicians, decides to open a new practice in the same community as the employer's practice. Upon opening this practice, the two referring physicians continue to refer to this physical therapist, regardless of the new office location. The new practitioner is directly competing with his past employer and is using previously gained contacts and information at the expense of the former employer's practice. If a restrictive covenant were in place, the employee could be violating the contract by opening a new practice in the same vicinity. However, the rules and regulations concerning restrictive covenants vary from state to state.

Restrictive covenants have been challenged in the courts. For the most part, if the restrictive covenant is reasonable, it will stand the test of a court action.

It is important to realize that employees who leave a private practice usually do not have the funds for a legal action, so the restrictive covenant serves to prevent the situation from arising. Restrictive covenants usually apply to a limited time period and to a limited geographic area in which the employee is prohibited from working after leaving the private practice.

Attorneys draft the terms of the agreement in legal format. Frequently, after a private practice develops an employment agreement with the aid of its attorney, it uses this agreement for all employees filling similar positions.

Negotiations

Throughout the life of the private practice, business negotiations are required in many situations. This is an area in which the corporation's attorney may prove to be very important, as attorneys are skilled in negotiating contracts and other legal documents. Any time that the practice enters into a legal arrangement, it is wise to use the attorney's services.

Lease

The first major area of negotiations is the office lease. The private practitioner can discuss the terms of the lease with the lessor (landlord). Since the lessor draws up the lease, it is skewed to the lessor's benefit. The corporation's attorney must review the lease and negotiate on the practice's behalf the best possible terms.

The lease protects the lessor and passes on all expenses possible to the tenants. Although this is the landlord's intent, the legal wording may make this unclear to persons not legally trained. The attorney can save the corporation considerable annoyance and money by thoroughly reviewing the lease.

Leases spell out many terms relating to the lessor and the lessee, including the parties engaged in the lease, the location of the leased property, the length of the lease, and the monthly rental. The lease also explains the rights of the lessor and the lessee, the method used to determine rent increases, and the insurance obligations of the lessee to protect the lessor's facility. Any additional information pertaining to the lease must be included or attached to the lease, which must be signed by both parties.

Negotiating with Outside Organizations

Practitioners should use the services of the attorney when entering into agreements with outside facilities, such as nursing homes. The attorney acts to protect the interests of the practice in these dealings, as well as in negotiating contracts with service companies, such as computer companies and servicing firms. The attorney protects the corporation in all litigation, knows how to resolve conflicts, and is employed to serve the practice's best interests.

One Final Note on the Attorney

The attorney has a smaller role after the start-up operations but should always be consulted if legal problems arise. After the start-up phase the attorney manages the corporation's minute books, may write new employee agreements when new employees are hired, and serves whenever the need arises.

However, it is important to remember that attorneys charge fees for their time, and the more their services are used, the higher the fees. Thus, when dealing with the attorney one should assume that "the meter is always running" and avoid wasting time. Moreover, attorneys frequently use subordinates to do some of their work. These people's services are less expensive, but they are also less qualified than the attorney hired for the practice. If errors arise from the work of the subordinates, their use may not prove to be cost-effective.

ATTORNEY CHECKLIST

	Date		*Date*
Conceptual advice		Legal Documentation (*cont'd*)	
Topic	___	Issuing stock	
Topic	___	certificates	___
Topic	___	Corporate annual	
		maintenance	___
		Employment	
Legal Documentation		agreements	___
Corporate name	___		
Articles of		Negotiations	
incorporation	___	Lease	___
Shareholders'		Outside organization	___
agreement	___	Outside organization	___
Buy-sell agreement	___	Outside organization	___
Ordering corporate			
seal and minute			
book	___		

ACCOUNTANT

The services of an accountant are more essential to the daily functioning of the physical therapy practice than are those of the attorney. The accountant's role may be minimal during the development phase, but as the practice becomes larger and more complex so does the accountant's role.

The accountant performs six primary services: assistance with loan acquisitions, development of a financial system, salary withholdings and tax payments, preparing financial statements, filing income tax returns, and financial planning.

Assistance with Loan Acquisitions

It is reasonable to consult an accountant before applying for a loan (see Ch. 3). The accountant can assist in calculations of projected revenues and expenses and can develop a formal presentation of these data for the loan officers. In addition, through experience in the community the accountant may be able to recommend a lending agency. An accountant with years of experience may even be able to supply the name of a lending officer.

Development of a Financial System

All businesses must have a flow of finances. One item that this requires is a method of writing and recording checks to an account or accounts payable. Another item is collecting payments from patients and recording them to patients' account or accounts receivable. Essentially, all financial matters will be organized through the accountant. The system chosen may be unfamiliar to a physical therapist, but will be second nature to the accountant.

Salary Withholdings and Tax Payments

In private practice the owners must pay wages to their employees and probably themselves. This may be the first time that payroll becomes their responsibility. The accountant instructs the new private practitioners how to write payroll checks with appropriate deductions for payroll taxes and Social Security (see Ch. 3). In addition to income tax and Social Security withholdings, the accountant instructs the owners how to make the correct withholding deposits. If these are not deposited in the bank, which acts as an agent for the government, financial penalties can be incurred. Additionally, the accountant, after reviewing the quarterly financial information, will instruct the owners if any quarterly tax payments must be made. The accountant will also complete the appropriate tax forms, which the owners sign and submit with the payments.

Financial Statements

The most important financial document is the balance sheet, or financial statement. The balance sheet provides an overview of the practice's financial position and summarizes its assets and liabilities, the difference between which is the net worth of the practice (see Ch. 9).

The statement of revenues lists all the revenues from various sources (different physical therapists and sale of supplies). The statement of operating expenses lists all expenses derived from all sources. The accurate difference between revenues and expenditures represents the profit or loss.

The various statements demonstrate financial trends in the practice and enable the owners to see how the business is performing. If revenues consistently drop over three quarters (9 months), the reason must be identified and remedial action undertaken.

Filing Income Tax Returns

Income tax returns for the private practice are different and usually more complicated to complete than personal tax returns. Depending on the practice's structure (sole proprietorship, partnership, or corporation) the accountant must comply with all regulations and file the appropriate tax returns.

Financial Planning

The accountant who has a good understanding of the private practice can prove valuable in financial planning. A profitable practice will benefit from tax planning and achieve tax savings. An accountant familiar with the private practice and the current tax laws can help the owners to prosper. For example, income paid to owners and employees as salaries and classified as expenses (such as travel expenses for continuing education and lunches brought into the office for the staff) are nontaxable. Professional association dues and license fees are expenses to the business and are paid with pretax dollars. This benefits the individual therapists, who otherwise would have to pay these dues and fees with after-tax dollars. Large-scale financial planning includes pension plans, profit sharing, tax-sheltered investments, estate planning, and tax planning.

One Final Note on the Accountant

Accountants charge for their time and their fee is usually quite high. Like attorneys, accountants frequently delegate some of their tasks to subordinates, whose hourly fee may be less than those of the accountant. Any clerical work that can be done within the practitioners' office reduces the accountant's time, which will prove cost-effective to the practice. The way that the practice uses the services of the accountant can have either a positive effect (e.g., the practice may be enabled to expand and become more complex) or a negative effect (e.g., if the materials needed by the accountant are not efficiently prepared).

ACCOUNTANT CHECKLIST

	Date
Assistance with loan acquisition	_____
Development of financial system	_____
Salary withholdings and tax payments	_____
Financial statements	_____
Filing income tax returns	_____
Financial Planning	_____
Topic	_____
Topic	_____
Topic	_____

LOAN OFFICER

The loan officer of the lending institution helps the private practice secure the initial loan by discussing the various types of available loans and the ramifications of each type with the client (see Ch. 3). This officer can also be helpful to the practice after it becomes successful, since additional funds for expansion may be needed. The development of a credit line may provide backup funds for the practice. Therefore, a cooperative loan officer may prove helpful both when opening and while operating a practice.

INSURANCE AGENT

Upon opening a private practice there are three mandatory and three optional types of insurance to purchase. The mandatory policies are professional liability, office liability, and workers' compensation; the optional policies are disability, disability buy-sell, and life.

Mandatory Policies

Professional liability insurance protects the owners in the event that they are sued for malpractice. There are two major forms of this type of coverage, occurrence and claims-made. Occurrence coverage protects the firm as long as the insurance was in force when the alleged incident occurred. If a lawsuit is brought against the practice three years after the incident and one year after the practice was closed, this type of policy would still provide protection. Claims-made coverage protects the practice if the coverage is in effect when the claim is made. If the alleged incident occurred three years before and the claims-made policy was terminated one year before the lawsuit, this coverage would not protect the practice. However, claims-made policies usually allow for the purchase of a "tail" when the policy ends, which allows coverage for practices that no longer exist.

Insurance carriers will offer one or the other type of insurance and market their policies based upon the advantages provided by each type. Increases in annual premiums are frequently downplayed but they obviously occur. The insurance coverage required is another issue to resolve when evaluating the cost of the insurance premiums. In today's litigious society the more insurance coverage, the better, since financial awards for malpractice claims are often exorbitant. It is common to obtain insurance coverage for liability limits of $1 million/$3 million which provides coverage for $1 million for any single occurrence and $3 million for any 12-month period.

Office liability insurance protects the private practice office from damage to the physical facility. If equipment or carpeting is stolen or damaged by flood, this policy would replace the stolen or damaged goods. This coverage also protects the practice against claims for personal injury occurring on the premises.

Workers' compensation insurance covers the private practice for expenses associated with the medical bills of employees who are injured on the job.

Optional Policies

Disability insurance covers the policyholder in the event of a disabling injury resulting in inability to work. Generally the owner of a private practice cannot afford to lose income over a period of time because of an injury. Disability insurance provides a monthly income during the period of disability. The key to policies of this nature is the carrier's definition of disability; the policy whose definition maximally protects the private practitioner is the policy of choice. Such a policy should prevent disagreements and the possibility of no payment if the insurance company challenges the claim.

Disability buy-sell insurance covers the owners of a private practice if one of the owners becomes disabled and is no longer able to take part in the practice. This policy provides the necessary funds to buy the disabled owner's shares of stock. Life insurance provides for financial protection of policyholder's family in the event of death.

A multitude of policies with varying coverages and premiums are available. When investigating insurance coverage for the private practice, the choices may seem extremely complicated. An insurance agent can help the private practitioner determine the practice's specific insurance needs and recommend which policies to purchase. Usually the higher the coverage the higher the premiums. New private practices must purchase the mandatory insurance policies but may defer purchase of the optional policies until the practice can afford the premiums.

INSURANCE CHECKLIST

Date Purchased

Professional liability   ———

Office liability   ———

Workers' compensation   ———

Disability   ———

Disability buy-sell   ———

Life   ———

BUSINESS SYSTEMS REPRESENTATIVE

When the private practice opens, a business system must be in place. A business systems representative is able to identify the specific needs of the practice and determine the system required. The basic business system includes patient ledger cards, a daily record of charges and receipts, a check writing mechanism, and a payroll and disbursement journal.

The patient ledger card provides space for recording specific patient information, including name, address, telephone number, referral source, treating physical therapist, dates of visits, description of services provided, and itemized charges for services. Any payments received for these services or any prior services are recorded, as are any adjustments to the fees charged. The last item on the card is the balance due following each visit.

The daily record of charges and receipts is a method of processing all patients treated on a given day on one form. A common method is the one-step entry, which facilitates data entry on the ledger card and the daily record of charges and receipts. This form of recording also permits daily computation of the accounts receivable. Another advantage of this system is that it provides documentation of fees generated and revenues collected by each therapist.

The check writing system is nothing more than a checkbook used solely for the business. This checkbook should be of the kind that provides a carbon copy or stub for ease of record keeping. The check should also have space for describing where the funds were spent. The check carbons or stubs should have space for payroll deductions so that employees may know the amounts of income tax and Social Security withholdings. These checks are frequently produced by the business systems representative. Before ordering them the private practitioner must obtain a specification sheet from the bank to ensure that the checks will follow the bank's system.

The payroll and disbursement journal is a method of processing all the checks written by the business. When the checks are written, the information is entered in this journal, which allows all checks to be written on one form and allows all items of similar type to be organized in spreadsheet fashion. Accordingly, the expenditures of the private practice can be clearly followed by inspection of this journal.

BUSINESS SYSTEMS REPRESENTATIVE CHECKLIST

Date Initiated

Ledger cards   _____

Daily record of charges
and receipts   _____

Check writing system   _____

Payroll and
disbursement journal   _____

COMPUTER REPRESENTATIVE

The private practice's computer representative advises the owners on their computer needs. Although it is quite possible to open the private practice without computers, at some time consideration of computerization will arise. The computer representative will evaluate the practice with respect to items such as number of patients, number of treatments per patient, number of payments received, number of checks written, and type of written communications. Following an assessment of the practice's needs, the computer representative will present a plan for computerization, including recommendations for choosing computer hardware and software. In selecting hardware the speed and memory of the computer, the keyboard, and the quality of the printer should be considered. The software may include a patient billing package and a word processing program. The practitioners may decide to lease or purchase the computer package or to hire a company to perform some or all of the necessary computer tasks (see Ch. 12).

EQUIPMENT SALESPERSON

As soon as word is out that a new private physical therapy practice has been established in the community, equipment sales representatives will contact the owners. All representatives will try to show how their product is better than the competitors'. All equipment should be evaluated before purchasing, and the advantages and disadvantages of purchasing from one company or spreading the purchases around to many companies should be considered. Moreover, all capital equipment prices are negotiable. Since the markup on capital equipment is very high, most equipment salespersons are willing to lower the price somewhat, perhaps by 20 percent, to close a sale.

Salespeople can help the practice in certain situations. They can lend equipment on a trial basis until a decision is made on which product to purchase. They can also supply equipment or replacement parts when something breaks. Even if one company receives most of the practice's business, the practitioners should always remain in contact with other companies, which will enhance their ability to negotiate prices and also keeps them in a position to buy from the various salespeople.

PHYSICAL THERAPY SUPPLIES SALESPERSON

The physical therapy supplies salesperson is frequently the same person as the equipment sales representative. However, some equipment companies sell only capital equipment and not physical therapy supplies. Once the private practitioner knows who sells and stocks which products and arranges for services, the efficiency of the practice will be increased.

OFFICE SUPPLIES SALESPERSON

The practice will need to find a local office supply company, preferably one that will allow telephone orders and will deliver on the same day.

Attorney

Name: Address: Phone #:

Accountant

Name: Address: Phone #:

Loan Officer

Name: Address: Phone #:

Insurance Agent

Name: Address: Phone #:

Business Systems Representative

Name: Address: Phone #:

Computer Representative

Name: Address: Phone #:

Equipment Salesperson

Name: Address: Phone #:

Physical Therapy Supplies Salesperson

Name: Address: Phone #:

Office Supplies Salesperson

Name: Address: Phone #:

Professional Colleagues

Name: Address: Phone #:

Name: Address: Phone #:

Name: Address: Phone #:

Family and Friends

Name: Address: Phone #:

Name: Address: Phone #:

Name: Address: Phone #:

Fig. 4-1. Support systems directory.

PROFESSIONAL COLLEAGUES

Fellow health professionals can prove very important to the growth and development of the new private practice. Through discussion with professional colleagues, practitioners are able to keep abreast of the changing health care environment. This network can prove most valuable to the practice.

FAMILY AND FRIENDS

As is true for all privately held businesses, in a new private practice one must leave the 9-to-5 work mentality behind. The time and energy commitments needed to build a private practice are very great and detract from time and energy typically spent elsewhere, often with the family. The practitioner's family should know of the time and energy requirements in advance and must be willing to sacrifice during the development of the practice. Hopefully, once the practice is functioning smoothly and profitably, the private practitioner can restructure these time and energy commitments and thereby give more time and attention to family and friends.

SUMMARY

This chapter discusses the many support systems necessary for a successful private practice. At different stages of the practice's development some of these systems will be more important than others. Members of the support systems include persons who will have an impact on the development and maintenance of the business as well as those who are of primary importance to the owners' lives.

SUGGESTED READINGS

Brimer MA: Fundamentals of Private Practice in Physical Therapy. Charles C Thomas, Springfield, IL, 1988

Butler KG (ed): Prospering in Private Practice—A Handbook for Speech-Language Pathology and Audiology. Aspen Publishers, Rockville, MD, 1986

Deaton C: Your Private Practice. Vol. 3. Financial Planning. Ben E. Johnston, Jr. & Peter J. Lord, Lake City, FL, 1982

Greene GG: How to Start and Manage Your Own Business. 3rd Ed. New American Library, New York, 1987

J.K. Lasser Tax Institute: How To Run A Small Business. 6th Ed. McGraw-Hill, New York, 1989

Johnston BE, Lord PJ: Your Private Practice. Vol. 2. Planning and Organization. Ben E. Johnston, Jr. & Peter J. Lord, Lake City, FL, 1982

Sokol S: Your Insurance Advisor. Barnes & Noble Books, New York, 1977

St. Paul Fire and Marine Insurance Company: Claims-made insurance: Its impact on PPS members. Whirlpool 8(4):42–43, 1985

Young CR: Making Your Practice Grow—a Useful Guide for the Health Care Professional. Bracey Publishing Co., Farmington Hills, MI, 1984

5

LOCATION OF THE PRIVATE PRACTICE

The location of the physical therapy practice is critical to its success. New practitioners must do a considerable amount of investigation before choosing a location.

CHOICE OF THE COMMUNITY

Desired Life-Style

Rural Community

The idea of living in a rural rather than an urban community is very appealing to many people. However, when choosing a rural community, physical therapists are accepting a smaller population base on which to draw, as well as fewer physicians and smaller hospitals. Therefore, in a rural community the physical therapist needs to be a generalist rather than a specialist. Since there are fewer physical therapists in the community, each practicing therapist must treat all types of patient problems.

Physical therapists in rural settings must realize the importance of becoming involved in the community in ways other than their patient care responsibilities. Knowing people on a personal basis is very important in rural communities. Community involvement is a valuable method for the new practitioner to become known and develop a successful private practice.

Urban Community

The rural community is not for everyone. Those who prefer the urban setting are selecting more populated communities with more physical therapists, more physicians, and more hospitals, including many general hospitals and others that provide specialized services. An urban community permits physical therapists to specialize, as there are others to provide the alternative services. Private practitioners in urban communities may select the type of practice they want even though competition for the patient care market is greater.

In addition to their patient care responsibilities, physical therapists may choose to become involved in community activities. Although such involvement may prove helpful in an urban setting, it is probably not nearly as critical for the success of the practice as it is for the rural physical therapist, since larger communities are less personal.

Personal Factors

It is important to consider the personal needs and desires of the therapist's immediate family. Some of these needs may be related to cost of living, type of housing, availability of schools, climate, size of the community, and religious affiliation. It is important to investigate whether the family is compatible with the surroundings before opening a private practice.

Frequently the opening of a private practice does not require relocation of the family unit. In this case a major personal issue may be one of economics. When starting a private practice the practitioner frequently will earn less for many months or years. The financial impact of this on the family unit must be addressed beforehand. Sometimes entering private practice must be delayed until family obligations are fulfilled.

Characteristics of the Community

The community to be served must be investigated before opening a private practice. Population characteristics, general economy, level of the health care community, professional competition, and health care providers must be considered. All will have a bearing on the potential growth of the practice.

Population Characteristics

The demographics of the community must be considered. If the community is composed mainly of heavy-industry laborers, the practitioner can expect to treat work-related injuries. This type of patient population may be a positive or negative factor depending upon the Workers' Compensation reimbursement policy of the state. Every state has specific regulations concerning payment of Workers' Compensation claims. Moreover, the required paperwork may prove to be a nuisance. However, if the goal of the practice is to promote functional capacity evaluation and work hardening, this population may prove to be ideal.

If the community is composed largely of elderly persons, the private practitioner can expect to treat patients on Medicare. This has considerable impact as the federal government has imposed strict limits on the amount of Medicare reimbursement for outpatient physical therapy. However, as of the late 1980s, if the private practice is a certified rehabilitation agency, the dollar limit is not as rigid, but the paperwork is greater.

If the community is primarily composed of young, healthy, athletic individuals, the practice can expect to treat athletic injuries, as young people frequently participate in a variety of athletic activities during their leisure time.

If the community is composed of people of a foreign culture and language, the private practice can expect to treat culturally different people. This will not affect the type of patient problems treated but may affect staffing policies. It may be imperative to have a physical therapist or secretarial staff member who is bilingual to facilitate communication concerning patient scheduling and treatment.

General Economy

The general economy will have a significant impact on the private practice. If factory workers are being laid off, there will be a decrease in work-related injuries. In another patient population, elderly persons who are not affluent may not be able to afford therapy after the Medicare limit has been met. This creates the ethical dilemma of whether to continue to treat patients for no reimbursement or to discharge patients before they are fully rehabilitated.

In an affluent community the practitioner would rightly be led to believe that money is generally available and therefore that patients should be able to pay their medical and physical therapy bills. Moreover, many wealthier patients receive physical therapy for problems that they do not consider major. People whose insurance does not provide coverage for physical therapy may choose not to attend physical therapy sessions. Poorer people with insurance may not be able to afford their portion of the bill. The practitioner must choose either to accept partial payment for services rendered or to provide services only for full payment.

Professional Level of the Health Care Community

The level of the health professional community must be investigated. The quality and type of services provided in the local hospitals may be geared to various types of patient problems. Hospitals may provide care for unique problems or specialized care not normally available. This may serve to raise the level of professionalism in the health care community and may also raise the quality of services provided by the local physicians and other health care providers.

If the private practice plans to provide a unique rehabilitation service, there must be a need for such a service within the professional community. The health care community must be aware of the service to refer patients to the practice. If the practice offers a service not congruent with the health care community, referrals will not be generated. If the service is ahead of its time, it may be difficult to market.

Competition

The growing number of physical therapy private practices is a double-edged sword. One view is that more such practices means greater visibility and greater respect from the public. This furthers public awareness of the profession. Increased awareness of the need for physical therapy services on the part of both health care professionals and potential patients is a plus. On the other hand, private practices in the same community will be vying for the same patient market. This may lead to too many private practices with too few patients to treat.

Therefore, new private practitioners must investigate who the other private practitioners are. This serves many purposes:

1. To confirm that a private practice can exist in the community
2. To assess the clinical and professional skills of the other practitioners so that the new practice can provide services that complement those of the existing practices and fill community needs
3. To avoid locating too close to existing practices, which would create direct competition for patients from the same referral sources and geographic areas
4. To identify referral sources that use the existing physical therapy practices and also those that do not
5. To seek assistance from the existing practitioners that can help to minimize the number of errors made in the new practice.

Health Care Providers

Besides physical therapists, there are many health care providers who compete for the same patients. Investigating these other health care providers further improves the understanding of the community. Who these providers are, what services they offer, and how they generate referrals constitute some of the information desired.

Doctors of chiropractic medicine are gaining respect from health care consumers. Although they still emphasize treatment for spinal dysfunction, chiropractors are treating patients with various types of problems. Chiropractors are increasing their use of physical therapy modalities, and they may often compete with physical therapists for the same patient. However, there are many areas in which the two can work together to enhance the quality of patient care.

Massage therapists frequently ally themselves with chiropractors. These therapists specialize in the use of therapeutic massage, on which, for the most part, they rely to a far greater extent than do physical therapists. While massage therapists work the soft tissue, chiropractors are more apt to move vertebrae.

Athletic trainers are gradually increasing their education, clinical skills, and areas of employment. In the past athletic trainers worked only with sports teams, but as of the late 1980s they are starting to work alongside physicians and physical therapists. This relationship provides well-rounded prevention and rehabilitation programs in sports-related facilities. However, in many of these facilities athletic trainers and physical therapists are carrying out essentially the same clinical responsibilities.

OBTAINING REFERRALS

The prospective private practitioner must do an excellent job of market research to choose the correct location. One of the key elements in this process is to identify and obtain information about the potential referral system.

Referral-for-Profit Arrangements

During the 1980s the American Physical Therapy Association addressed the controversial issue of referral for profit. This concept was initially called physician-owned physical therapy services (POPTS), the implication being that the physical therapists were working for the physicians. This issue was hotly debated. Those who took the negative view felt the referrals to physical therapists were made for the sole purpose of financial remuneration and that working for physicians undermined the profession of physical therapy. The other side of the argument was that the arrangement promotes a close and educational interaction with the referring physician, which improves the ability to treat orthopedic and sports medicine patients. The controversy over this issue went on for years. The issue of POPTS gradually moved to the broader issue of all referral-for-profit arrangements as many states passed laws against any form of fee splitting or financial remuneration for referrals.

A different type of referral-for-profit arrangement, viewed as a joint venture, became the new way for physicians to be reimbursed financially for referring patients to physical therapists. Through a corporation formed among physicians and physical therapists, the physicians refer patients primarily to a jointly owned rehabilitation facility. Instead of being paid for the referral, the physician profits from the success of the rehabilitation facility. Many different variations of referral-for-profit concept are being practiced in the United States.

Regardless of one's view of this controversial issue, its importance to new private practices must be understood. A physician who has a financial interest in a specific physical therapy clinic may be expected to refer patients primarily to that clinic. A new practice in this community should not expect referrals from such physicians. If many physicians choose to enter into such relationships in one community, the number of available referral sources decreases. These arrangements induce physicians to refer to specific physical therapy clinics on the basis of financial benefit, which unfortunately seems to be more important to some, but not all, physicians than quality of care. However, those physicians who do not wish to tie themselves to a specific clinic are concerned about quality care, advanced clinical skills, and patient convenience.

Knowing the referral arrangements that exist in various communities will allow the private practitioner to choose the office location that is best in terms of geographic desirability and availability of referrals. It is important to avoid opening the practice close to physicians known to have referral arrangements. Location at a distance of 5 to 10 miles or in a different city or county may make a major difference for a private practice. Physicians in the new community who are not in a referral-for-profit arrangement are potential referral sources. In addition, physicians who have such arrangements in other communities, cities, or counties, even a few miles away, may refer to the new practice those patients who live near the new facility and do not wish to commute to the physician's clinic.

Determining if the Services Are Needed

When selecting a community one important question is: Is there a need for a physical therapy private practice? This question may have many answers that justify opening the new practice. However, it is imperative that it be answered affirmatively before proceeding.

If there is a shortage of nonhospital outpatient physical therapy services, then opening a practice may be a good idea. A nonhospital private practice allows for a pleasant environment catering to the needs of the patients. The outpatient with a fractured elbow does not have to share a mat table with a semiconscious neurologic patient. Moreover, the private practice can accommodate the community's needs concerning hours of operation, including early morning, late evening, and weekend coverage.

The quality of care or specialty service provided may be further advanced than the state-of-the-art community services. If this is true, opening the practice is a good idea. A service that represents higher quality or advanced level becomes a salable commodity.

If the new practitioners are highly respected in the community, this may generate referrals. The development of a sound community reputation through either prior hospital employment or university affiliation is a plus. It is possible to assess the potential for referrals from previously established relationships.

Starting a new practice in a community may not be feasible if avenues of referrals are not available. If a community has too many physical therapy services for its size, opening a new facility may prove very risky. For unknown practitioners in a congested physical therapy community it may take longer to develop a referral base than financial resources allow.

Community Grapevine

When a new physical therapy practice opens in a community, the unofficial health professional network can help the practice by serving as a good source of publicity. Physical therapists who respect the new practice are able to enlighten referral sources about the facility and the services available there. Through the goodwill of fellow professionals the new practice may flourish. In addition, allies are usually willing and able to share their experiences and save the new practitioners some of the growing pains.

On the other hand, nothing can hurt a new practice as much as enemies in the health professional network. Negative information that precedes the opening of a new practice may prove insurmountable. Because changing a negative reputation—a necessary prelude to cultivating a positive image—may prove impossible, negative information may close the door to any opportunity.

New private practitioners should strive for a positive reputation concerning all facets of their professional and personal lives throughout the life of the practice. Essentially, the golden rule of treating others as one wishes to be treated by them may serve physical therapists well during their careers. One cannot predict future career directions and the consequent need for health professional allies.

Private Practice Location Checklist

	Notes
Desired life-style	———
Personal factors	———
Population characteristics	———
General economy	———
Professional level of health care community	———
Competition	———
Health care providers	———
Referral-for-profit arrangements	———
Need for the services	———
Community grapevine	———

OFFICE SITE

Many considerations enter into the decision of where to set up office. Physical location, accessibility and safety, and parking, are some of these factors. The possibility of sharing office space with another health care provider should also be considered.

Physical Location

The importance of a nearby medical complex must be considered. If the office is near a medical complex, potential patients are more likely to know the location of the office. In addition, proximity to a medical complex may bring in referrals through friendly relationships with hospital employees. Physical therapists at the hospital may send their overflow patients to the new practice, and the office buildings near hospitals will certainly have physicians' offices, which places the new practice near potential referral sources.

If the practice's office is not near a medical complex, the area may be less congested and more accessible to patients. Furthermore, if the referral sources are geographically scattered, being near a hospital complex may not be important.

Accessibility and Safety

When selecting the office site for the private practice, the location should be considered from the patients' perspective. For those who drive to the office, the drive has to be convenient, that is, the roads to the office must not be congested because of construction, traffic, or school zones. For patients who do not drive, public transportation must be available. Ease of accessibility for patients who use wheelchairs or ambulatory assistive devices is essential.

Another important issue is the neighborhood in which the office is located. Patients do not like to visit offices in high-crime areas. The private practice must be able, with minimal inconvenience, to accommodate the needs of the patients. Any factor that might deter patients from coming for physical therapy must be overcome.

Parking

Parking can create major difficulties for private practices. There must be enough parking spaces for the patients of the health care providers in the building in which the office is located. Some buildings assign a specific number of parking spaces to each office; others do not, and patients complain when spaces are not available. In large buildings with a limited number of spaces, the number of staff personnel in each tenant's office should be investigated. Office personnel frequently occupy many of the parking spaces provided for patients unless there are rules against this. Handicapped parking spaces are essential and should be clearly marked.

If there is a parking fee, determining who pays it may be an important decision. Patients do not appreciate having to pay for parking in addition to paying for physical therapy services. It may be possible for the private practice to pay the parking expense for their patients. This payment may even be made on a monthly basis or may be included in the monthly rental. A building with an excess of available parking to allow for growth of the practice and with no parking fee would be ideal.

Sharing Office Space

Sharing office space with another health care practitioner may be one way to ease the burden of starting in private practice. Sharing space permits reduction in office operating expenses through savings on rent, electricity, water, telephones, office personnel, and office furnishings. An additional benefit is the visibility of the physical therapy practice to patients of the other health care provider.

The disadvantage of sharing is that the physical therapy provider loses some control over the office, as the other health care practitioner will have a voice in all decisions affecting both practices.

OFFICE SITE CHECKLIST

Physical location   _____

Accessibility and safety   _____

Parking   _____

Sharing office space   _____

SUMMARY

This chapter discusses many issues that must be considered when deciding where to locate a new private practice, including personal preferences, community population, economic considerations, and the health care community. Elements necessary for patient convenience in deciding on the office site are also identified.

SUGGESTED READINGS

Bartlett RC: The physician-physical therapist financial arrangement. Whirlpool 8(4):35–40, 1985

Butler KG (ed): Prospering In Private Practice—A Handbook For Speech-Language Pathology And Audiology. Aspen Publications, Rockville, MD, 1986

Castle DE: Growth through joint ventures. Whirlpool 10(4):42–44, 1987

Johnston BE, Lord PJ: Your Private Practice. Vol. 2. Planning And Organization. Ben E. Johnston Jr. & Peter J. Lord, Lake City, FL, 1982

Naso A: A close look at POPTS practices in New Jersey. Whirlpool 10(1):44–48, 1987

Snook ID, Kaye EM: A Guide To Health Care Joint Ventures. Aspen Publications, Rockville, MD, 1987

Young CR: Making Your Practice Grow—A Useful Guide for the Health Care Professional. Bracey Publishing Co., Farmington Hills, MI, 1984

6

PLANNING, DESIGN, AND CONSTRUCTION OF THE PHYSICAL FACILITY

One of the best investments that a private practitioner can make is a distinctively designed office. This should be a high-priority item for many reasons. First, the appearance of the office is an important factor in promoting the practice. It is one of the main criteria patients use in judging the quality of services provided. Offering professional services in an environment that is comfortable and reassuring to the patient is an essential part of a promotional program. The office leaves lasting impressions with the patient and family. Second, the efficiency of the staff depends on providing a proper environment for patient care.

This chapter offers a practical approach to creating an appropriate physical therapy environment for a private practice. Checklists and charts are included to provide a foundation for decision making.

As in any other undertaking, the personal time and effort put into the project is directly proportional to the satisfaction with the results. Private practitioners should take their time in the process of planning, design, and construction. Solutions and alternatives that may not be common in physical therapy should be considered. Looking at everybody else's office and copying the layout is not the best way to design an office or a practice. A consumer-oriented focus will result in an improved design. There is rarely only one correct decision. The decision should be based on what is best for the individual practitioner and the intended patient population.

ADVANCE PLANNING FOR THE OFFICE DESIGN

During the planning process the ideal state is first defined and the plan is then modified, redefined, and brought to a practical level. The following steps are typical of the planning process:

Step 1. Determine the characteristics of the population to be served
Step 2. Establish the profile of physicians within a geographic radius
Step 3. Determine the tentative services to be provided
Step 4. Project the expected volume
Step 5. Project staffing requirements
Step 6. Determine major equipment requirements
Step 7. Determine special space needs
Step 8. Determine anticipated growth of the practice
Step 9. Determine the public image to be created or supported
Step 10. Determine the cost

Putting time and effort into the above determinations will be of major assistance in creating the optimal office design and will provide the basis for sound decisions.

Sources of Free Information

Numerous people, organizations, companies, and places are potential sources of information for designing an office. The limiting factor is how much time and energy the practitioner has available. The first experience in designing office space will take more time than subsequent office moves. Previous office design experience in a private practice setting will provide a wealth of information and decrease the time needed for the project.

A surprising amount of information can be obtained at little or no cost:

1. Chambers of commece are excellent sources of information about types of firms, numbers and skills of employees, wages, community demographics, and other data.
2. The U.S. Health Systems Agency (HSA) provides information regarding community health services and needs, facilities, and personnel.
3. The American Physical Therapy Association prints an annual buying guide and several bibliographies pertaining to different facets of design.
4. It is helpful to photograph other physical therapy offices and to interview the therapists regarding what they would do differently if they had it to do over again.

Physicians, patients, staff, architects, other health care providers, and the private practitioner can make invaluable contributions to the planning process. Information may be obtained by personal interviews, telephone conversations, written requests, visiting different practices in different locations, and asking questions of colleagues.

Hiring Consultants

Since the most difficult and expensive decisions are made early in the process, hired consultants and experts should be decided on as early as feasible. Choosing the right consultants can mean the difference between success and failure.

Architect

The architect's role in designing an office involves a great deal more than making a blueprint and will be determined by the agreement made with the landlord. A landlord who pays the fees will define the architect's responsibilities; a private practitioner who pays the fees will contract the individual services needed. In either case the architect is responsible for fully detailed architectural and mechanical work drawings and specifications, as well as for meeting all local building codes and zoning restrictions and for supplying samples of materials suggested for use in construction. Optionally, the architect may negotiate with contractors, suggest cheaper construction methods, and act as liaison between the private practitioner and the contractor. Therefore the interview with the architect must be extensive and provide the following information:

1. Professional fees by the hour or by the project (hourly fees average between $100 and $150)
2. Photographs of past work
3. Evidence of communication style compatible with that of the practitioner
4. Recommendations/references
5. Addresses of previous projects to be visited

Interior Decorator

The interior decorator is responsible for creating the intended atmosphere of the office through the use of color, fabric, furniture, floor covering, accessories, and wall hangings. The physical atmosphere is a major part of the total image.

The qualifications of decorators vary. Decorators may be independent contractors or may be employed by a furniture store or supplier. The independent decorators generally belong to the American Society of Interior Designers and may use the initials ASID following their names. Requirements for membership in ASID are stringent; the members are tested and have to submit portfolios with pictures of their previous work.

ASID decorators generally charge by the hour ($50 to $150) or by the project. If the charge is by the project, a fee must be negotiated in advance and a contract drawn up. A retainer must be paid and a major part of the fee withheld until the office has been completed satisfactorily. The advantages of hiring ASID decorators is that they have a greater level of expertise and they make their purchases from a wide range of manufacturers since their expenditures will not affect their professional fees.

Interior decorators affiliated with a furniture store or major supplier do not charge a professional fee. However, their main interest is to sell their store's merchanidse exclusively because their only fee is the commission they make on such sales.

Both types of interior decorator should provide the following services:

1. Space planning
2. Design presentation through drawings and photographs

3. Samples of materials to be used
4. Troubleshooting and negotiations from purchase to installation

Equipment Representatives

Major equipment manufacturers and suppliers have sales representatives who are knowledgeable about space planning. Their advice is a courtesy to those customers who are planning to purchase equipment through their companies. Although the primary interest of these experts is to sell their company's equipment, they can be of assistance in placing equipment in the most advantageous locations within the office suite. In addition, they will provide installation templates for their equipment and a great deal of information regarding what is being done by other physical therapists within the area.

Narrative Proposal

Following the preliminary investigation, a clear, easily understood statement of what the practice will involve is required. This statement will be provided to the architect and any other designated experts to assist in the design of the office space.

The proposal should include the following information, which will lead to the decision of how much space will be required:

1. Expected patient volume
2. Staff requirements
3. Anticipated growth
4. Equipment of major size
5. Any special space requirements
6. Total office space requirements

The initial estimate of office space required will also be included in the proposal.

Estimating Space Requirements

A preliminary estimate of total space required is needed for the budget process and for suite selection. This will be reassessed when the architect prepares the preliminary blueprints. Most first-time private practitioners underestimate space requirements to keep initial overhead down, disregarding anticipated future growth. This will prove to be an extremely costly mistake if 6 months later additional space is needed to handle current patient volume.

Figures 6-1 and 6-2 should be consulted for assistance in estimating required space from projected data on patient volume, staff, equipment, and services provided. These projections will help the practitoner to make an educated guess of how much space is needed. Individual practices may not need every designated room and might require some rooms not listed.

Step 1. Determine number of treatment rooms necessary to handle projected volume and staff.
 a. Divide available minutes of room use (office hours minus lunch multiplied

ROOM SPACE REQUIREMENTS				
Room	Suggested Dimensions	Required Square Footage	Units Required	Total Square Footage
Treatment Rooms (examples)	8' × 10' 9' × 9' 9' × 10'	80' 81' 90'	4 4 4	320' 324' 360'
Fitness Gym Area				

Hydrotherapy Room
  Small whirlpool
  Large whirlpool
  Lowboy whirlpool				

Waiting Room				
Business Office				
Staff Office				
Patient Bathroom				
Staff Bathroom				
Linen Laundry Room				
Storage				

Additional Areas
  Administrative office
  Conference room
  Biofeedback room
  Occupational therapy
  Speech therapy
  Computer room
  Isokinetic room				

Total Square Footage Needed = _____

Fig. 6-1. Worksheet for estimating space requirements for physical therapy office.

by 60) by total treatment time (treatment plus setup plus cleanup) in minutes to determine total number of patient visits per room per day.

$$\text{Patient visits room A} = \frac{\text{available time}}{\text{treatment time}}$$

b. Divide total projected visits (adjusted for visits not requiring treatment rooms) by number of visits produced by each room.

EQUIPMENT SPACE REQUIREMENTS					
Equipment Name	Quantity	Dimensions	Additional Space Needed	Fixed/ Unfixed	Special Needs
Mat Table (sample)	2	6' × 8'	Clearance All Sides	F	None

Total Square Footage Needed for Equipment = _____

Fig. 6-2. Worksheet for estimating space requirements for physical therapy equipment.

$$\text{Number of rooms needed} = \frac{\text{adjusted projected visits}}{\text{patient visits per room}}$$

Step 2. Determine size of fitness/gym area.
a. Add suggested space requirements of all major equipment.
b. Determine necessary wall space.
Step 3. Determine size of specialized treatment rooms (e.g., for hydrotherapy

room by using rough specifications from whirlpool manufacturers to determine space requirements of tanks).

Step 4. Determine the rooms and space necessary for non-patient care activities.

Step 5. Transfer information to Figure 6-1 and carry all numerical data across and down for an estimation of the total square footage of space needed.

PLANNING AND DESIGN SEQUENCE

Meeting with Leasing Agent

Most office complexes and buildings have a leasing agent, who can, be contacted by visiting the leasing office or calling the phone number given in the building directory or on an outside sign. This person usually represents the landlord throughout the leasing process until the lease is to be negotiated.

The leasing agent should show potential tenants all available space finished or unfinished, in the selected building. The practitioner should walk through all the leasable space regardless of the size of the suite. It is important to review each available suite regarding exposure, shape, natural lighting, and adjacent suites. If the suite has already been built out, it is necessary to visualize the amount of renovation that might be required.

The number of windows in the suite and their exposure—north, south, east, or west—will help the practitioner to estimate air conditioning and heating costs as well as the amount of natural lighting to expect throughout the day. The shape of the suite is critical in space planning. Odd shapes contribute to problems and require a really talented architect. The most desirable suites are rectangular or square.

It is important to note what suites are located on either side of the space under consideration to determine potential noise and traffic factors. For instance, being next door to a veterinarian on the ground floor may lead to problems with dog waste and barking. If an oddly shaped space is available adjacent to the suite being considered the landlord might be persuaded to include it at a discounted price.

When the tour of the available space and the building has been completed, the agent should supply the prospective tenant with a written description of the entire complex or building, including a complete list of tenants, total square footage, leased square footage, and local thoroughfares. In addition, the specifications of all the suites that the practitioner might consider and a blank copy of the lease used for closing should be requested. The former will be used to draw a preliminary layout, and the latter will be presented to the attorney at a later time.

Choosing the Desired Suite

All possible combinations of suites that will provide the approximate square footage that was initially estimated as required should be reviewed by the practitioner. The pros and cons of each of the potential suites should be listed and ranked according to their importance to determine the preferred or first choice of office space. Designation of a second choice is necessary in case the meeting with the landlord uncovers information previously omitted that would lead the practitioner to reconsider the first choice.

Meeting with the Landlord

It is not necessary for the attorney to be present at the first meeting with the landlord. The worksheet shown in Figure 6-3 should be used for this meeting, the purpose of which is to discuss issues such as length of lease, exclusive rights of providing physical therapy services, utilities and maintenance responsibilities, completion date of the suite, penalty clauses for delayed occupany, and who is going to pay for the construction or "build-out" of the suite. The latter issue can not be addressed until the architect creates the preliminary blueprints, which must include plumbing and electrical work.

The question of who pays the architect fees must be addressed. Any expense incurred before closing the lease might be wasted if the negotiations fail. In most instances the landlord will pay the architect's fees. However, a physical therapist unlike a physician, may not automatically be seen by the landlord as a desirable tenant. Leverage depends on how knowledgeable the landlord is regarding the potential earning power of a physical therapy office, the strength of the landlord's desire for tenants in general, the length of the lease, and how competitively the space is priced. Verbal or implied agreements should not be made at this time, aside from the question of the architect's fees, without the opinion of an attorney. Efforts to cut costs by not consulting an attorney may lead to a very costly and irreversible mistake.

Preparing a Preliminary Layout

It is advantageous to develop a preliminary office layout before the first meeting with the architect in order to obtain some perspective and to save architectural fees. Moreover, most architects have no idea of what the layout of a physical therapy office, should be. It is the responsibility of the practitioner to educate the architect regarding typical traffic flow, standard dimensions of specialty equipment, and the special needs of a physical therapy office. This will save time and improve the final design. The practitioner, not the architect, is the physical therapy expert and will have to live with any mistakes in design.

Two essential concepts to keep in mind during creation of the floor layout are function zones and traffic flow. *Function zones* are areas dedicated to a single major function, and each should work efficiently without adversely affecting another zone. For example, a hydrotherapy area would be considered a function zone and should be located where it would not interfere with another zone (e.g., the staff office). The practitioner should think about how the zones relate to one another and the locations at which they can interact most effectively.

The term *traffic patterns* or *flow* refers to how individuals get from one zone to the next. A desirable traffic pattern minimizes steps, considers safety, and

INITIAL MEETING WITH LANDLORD

Rent/Square Foot _____

Total Annual Rent _____   Monthly Rent _____

Length of Lease _____   Renewal Options _____

Option to Buy _____

Construction

    Architect fees _____

    Construction costs _____

    Carpet allowance _____

    Light fixture allowance _____

    Finishing allowance _____

    Signage costs _____

    Landlord representative _____

    Contractor used _____

    Option to use own contractor _____

    Anticipated completion date _____

    Penalty clause for late completion _____

Insurance _____

Taxes _____

Sublet _____

Maintenance Costs _____

Escalator Clause _____

    Request Copy of Standard Lease!

Fig. 6-3. Worksheet to be used during initial meeting with the landlord.

provides for maximum efficiency of office procedures.

It is useful at this stage to have handy a large pad of graph paper of ¼-inch scale, an architect's scale (a special ruler), tracing paper, scissors, erasers, and a large number of pencils. The dimensions supplied by the landlord should be used to create a shell of the suite that is as large as possible. Windows, doors, and any other fixtures (e.g., support columns) that must be part of the design should be included. Everything should be drawn to ¼-inch scale. Figure 6-4 represents the shell of a therapist-owned 3,200-square-foot office suite.

Two techniques can be used to prevent redesigning the basic shell or suite with every change in interior design. The first is to place tracing paper over the completed outline on the graph paper and sketch initial ideas on the tracing paper. The second is to use another sheet of graph paper to cut out the dimensions of the different furniture and equipment items that are to be included. This technique offers the opportunity to very quickly try out different placements of the equipment until the appropriate location has been found, at which time it is drawn directly on the graph paper.

Meeting with the Architect

The practitioner should be prepared with a wish list (prepared as if cost were no object), the narrative proposal, and ideas regarding a preliminary layout when meeting with the architect for the first time. The wish list will help clarify ideas and give the architect an understanding of what the practitioner desires. The more detailed the list, the better.

Review of the Final Blueprint

When meeting the architect to review the final blueprint, the practitoner should ask for an explanation of the symbols on the blueprint. The meeting should be scheduled when both parties are at their best and have adequate time. Once the blueprint is signed by the practitioner, it is very difficult to make changes. The blueprint will be referred to when disagreements arise during the construction phase; however any changes once construction begins are usually charged to the tenant unless the changes are necessary to meet local building codes.

Figure 6-5 is an example of the working blueprint. The practitioner should spend the needed extra time reviewing the blueprints, which should be provided to the practitioner several days before they are signed. Every function of the office should be visualized in every sequence. Every system, from administering an ultrasound treatment to photocopying of patient charts, should be "walked through" on the blueprint. If partners or office personnel have already been selected, they should be given the opportunity to walk through their prospective functions on the blueprint.

Second Meeting with the Landlord

It is advantageous to have an attorney present at the second meeting with the landlord to negotiate the lease. The practitioner should bring the partially completed worksheet (Fig. 6-3) to the meeting, at which both parties will have a copy of the completed blueprints. A decision must be made regarding which party is responsible for building and for paying office construction costs. If the practitioner/tenant is responsible for any portion of the work, an itemized break-

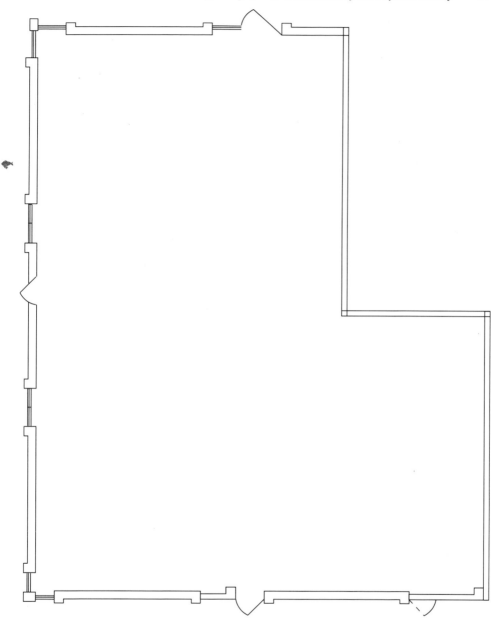

Fig. 6-4. The exterior shell of a therapist-owned 3,200-square-foot office suite.

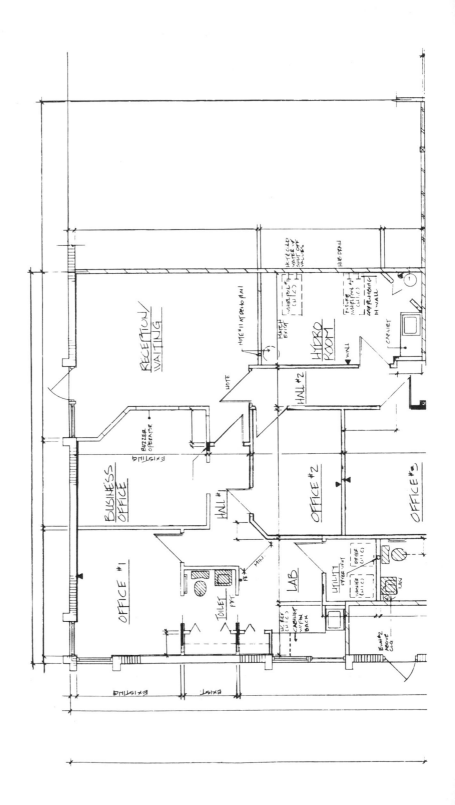

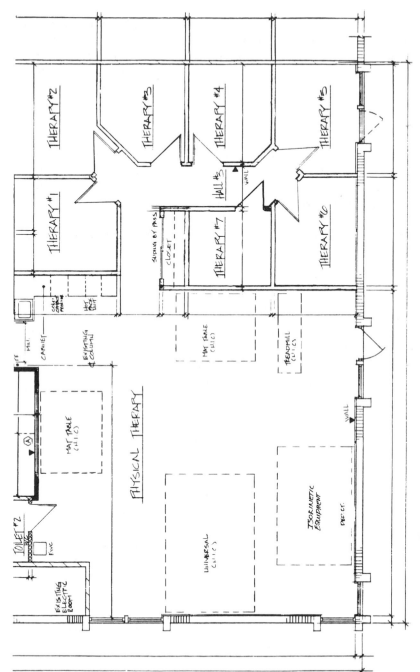

Fig. 6-5. An example of a working blueprint for a physical therapy office suite.

down and the total cost of the tenant's share must be included in the lease prior to signature. A work letter must be provided by the landlord itemizing in detail each party's obligations regarding construction. Consideration should be given to including a guaranteed date of completion as well as a performance clause. The landlord will then be financially penalized for failure to meet the deadline.

Submitting Negotiated Lease to Attorney

Ideally, an attorney should be included in the process by this point. It is a good idea to submit a blank copy of the lease to the attorney following the first meeting with the landlord. This will save time if the lease is so poor that the leasing effort must be abandoned or the lease must be completely rewritten. It is preferable that the attorney be present during the initial negotiations to avoid potential conflict. However, if no attorney has been part of the negotiations or has had an opportunity to review the lease, now is the time for one to examine the lease in minute detail.

Establishing an Estimated Budget

Before closing the lease, the projected budget for physically opening the office must be determined. The form shown in Figure 6-6 will aid in initial estimation of costs (Chapter 9 provides a thorough discussion of the budget process). The form in Figure 6-6 is suggested as a tool for determining the direct office opening expenses.

Closing of Lease

By the time of closing an attorney will have made the necessary changes, additions, and deletions to the lease in preparation for signature. At the closing the landlord is presented with a check for the negotiated security deposit and the first month's rent or whatever payments were negotiated. The practitioner would be ill advised to pay for any portion of the construction for which the tenant is responsible before its completion and inspection. Payment should be rendered only after the work has been completed to the practitioner's satisfaction.

MECHANICAL CONSIDERATIONS OF DESIGN
Lighting

A well selected lighting system enhances the environment and assists the physical therapist in carrying out appropriate treatment. Insufficient lighting and shadows are examples of problems. Natural lighting, when possible, adds a pleasant feeling to a room.

The system must be designed to meet code regulations and to be energy-efficient. It must be durable, have proper appearance, be maintained economically and easily, have the flexibility to permit additions if need be, and have a sufficent number of lighting zones.

LIGHTING CHECKLIST

Code requirements met   _____

Independent light   _____
switch for each room

Sufficient fixtures for   _____
optimal care and safety

Lighting zones energy-   _____
efficient and
economical

Spotlights for close   _____
examination (e.g.,
hydrotherapy for
wound care)

Sufficient natural   _____
lighting

Lighting fixtures   _____
aesthetically pleasing

Dimmer switches   _____
available for
appropriate treatment
rooms

Walls and Ceilings

The walls and ceilings are an essential component of the office's overall appearance. Both must be sturdy and pleasing to look at and require a minimal amount of maintenance. They must be strong enough to support the equipment that will be affixed to them. For example, walls built to code may not necessarily support the weight of a particular piece of equipment. If a ballet bar is provided for stretching, it must be anchored in a certain way.

The activity in physical therapy offices produces a great deal of noise, originating from the washer and dryer, whirlpool agitators, hot water heaters, dynamometers, and computer printers. The level of human noise depends on the number of patients in the gymnasium at one time and is increased by therapists who shout at their patients to kick harder on the isokinetic machine. The way to minimize acoustical problems is to consider the noise factor when laying out the floor plan and to incorporate noise minimizers in the walls, ceilings, and floors. Installation of sound-absorbing materials in the walls, background music piped in through the ceilings, and carpeting on the floors will minimize the noise.

Finally, ceiling requirements must be analyzed for height, energy efficiency

ESTIMATING COSTS FOR OPENING OFFICE

Lease

    Security deposit   _____

    First month's rent   _____

Professional Fees

    Attorney   _____

    Interior decorator   _____

Construction Costs

    Plumbing   _____

    Electrical   _____

    Lighting   _____

Finishing Interior

    Wallcovering   _____

    Floor covering   _____

    Window treatments   _____

    Art work   _____

    Plants   _____

    Patient pleasers   _____

Fig. 6-6. Worksheet for estimating costs of opening an office.

(continued)

Mirrors   _____

Furniture

  Business office   _____

  Reception area   _____

  Private office   _____

  Staff office   _____

  Misc.   _____

Utility Deposits

  Water   _____

  Electric   _____

  Phone   _____

Phone System   _____

Stereo System   _____

Security System   _____

Total   _____

Fig. 6-6. (*continued*)

and acoustics. Height is generally considered a given. However, if purchase of an autotraction table is planned, a higher ceiling than usual might be required.

WALL AND CEILING CHECKLIST

Sufficient privacy and   _____
damping of noise
through wall acoustics

Appropriate ceiling   _____
height to clear all
equipment

Reinforcement for   _____
equipment supported
by walls

Plumbing

Special attention must be devoted to the plumbing integrity of the office. Inadequate plumbing creates nightmares in patient care; insufficient hot water for the whirlpool bath and washing machine, stopped-up drains, and misplaced sinks all contribute to inefficient patient care. The architect must be provided with the manufacturer's complete plumbing specifications and rough-in drawings for any whirlpool equipment. These are readily available upon request from the manufacturer.

PLUMBING CHECKLIST

Floor drains canted and   _____
appropriately situated

Water valves and hose   _____
for cleaning tanks

Plumbing lines situated   _____
as close as possible to
one another

Hot water heater   _____
capacity adequate for
whirlpool and washing
machine volume
expected

Plumbing lines ¾-inch   _____
diameter or greater

PLUMBING CHECKLIST *continued*

Stainless steel sinks   _____   Height of sink and toilet   _____

Wheelchair-accessible   _____   fixtures ergonomically

bathroom   correct

Electrical Work

A viable electrical system with room for growth is the responsibility of a licensed electrician, who, along with the architect, must be provided with the electrical specifications of all equipment. It is a good idea to install dedicated lines for any major computer equipment or isokinetic equipment, with surge protectors to prevent disruption of services. Floor grounds and covered outlets in the hydrotherapy room are also recommended. Standard outlets are generally installed 12 inches off the floor, which can cause back strain to persons operating the equipment. Electricians should be instructed to place 36-inch-high outlets strategically throughout the office.

ELECTRICAL WORK CHECKLIST

Manufacturer's   _____   Light switches easily   _____
specifications met for   accessible
special equipment
                                                                        Fuse box accessible   _____

Outlets for treatment   _____
machines 36 inches off   Outlets located in a   _____
the floor   closet for installation of
                                                                        telephone system, radio
Outlets strategically   _____   system, and security
located throughout the   system
facility for every
possible piece of
equipment

Heating, Ventilation, and Air Conditioning

It is undesirable to provide one-zone heating, ventilation, and air conditioning (HVAC) in a physical therapy office regardless of the square footage. The temperature requirements of patients lying undressed in a treatment room, patients working out on the treadmill, and staff in the business office are distinctly different. If only one thermostat controls the entire office, nobody will be comfortable.

HVAC CHECKLIST

Vents located so that air does not directly blow on patients　_____

Enough individual HVAC zones to permit temperature control as required in the individual functional areas　_____

Location of excessively noisy fans and return ducts in low-traffic areas　_____

Vents in every treatment room　_____

Thermostats placed strategically and not under direct sunlight　_____

INSTALLED OFFICE SYSTEMS

Linen

A decision must be made regarding laundry handling before the final blueprints are drawn. Choices include using disposable paper goods, bringing linen home to wash, using a commercial service that picks up and delivers, or doing laundry in house.

If the decision is made to handle laundry in house, certain details have to be considered. A large-capacity commercial washer and dryer designed for energy conservation must be purchased. The washer and dryer must be located in an area close to the people who will be responsible for the laundry. Since these machines make considerable noise, the room has to be sound-proofed or located in an area that can function with a high sound level. The appropriate outlet, plumbing lines, vent for the dryer, and high-capacity hot water heater must be included in the blueprint. Finally, storage bins for clean and dirty laundry must be located throughout the office.

Security Systems

If the landlord does not supply a security system with the office suite, it is strongly recommended that one be installed. Physical therapists have expensive equipment, usually including computers, which may be removed by a burglar. The security system need not be installed during the construction phase of the project. There is an overabundance of security components that can be installed after the suite is finished and of companies to install them. However, an outlet should be provided in an accessible closet in which the main security panel will be located, since it requires electric power to function.

Telephone Systems

If installation of anything more than standard phones is planned, the telephone system should be considered during the construction phase. Computerized phone systems require a standard outlet for power and an additional outlet for a radio if piped-in music is to be provided when the hold button is in use. The control panel is generally located in an accessible storage closet, in which an outlet must be placed. Installation of multiple phones is made easier and cheaper if the conduits for the wiring and the boxes for phone jacks are roughed in by the electrician during construction.

Communication

It is advantageous to have some sort of intercom system to announce phone calls and arrival of patients so that the receptionist does not need to hand-carry every message. Most phone systems offer an intercom option so that a separate system is not necessary for communication within the office suite. If the decision is made to purchase a dedicated intercom system, the appropriate conduits, speakers, and outlets have to be roughed in during the construction phase.

Music

If it is decided to pipe in music via a built-in stereo system, the appropriate conduits, speakers and outlets, as well as a storage location for the amplifier, must be roughed in during the construction phase. Another alternative would be individual radios in the rooms that require music or a telephone system that will pipe in music through the phone speakers.

ROOM-BY-ROOM EVALUATION OF THE OFFICE DESIGN BEFORE AND AFTER CONSTRUCTION

All the key elements of the office design should be reviewed room by room both before and after construction. The appearance of the office should inspire the trust of its clients. The general goals regarding appearance should be met when the practitioner reviews the office.

Reception Area/Waiting Room

Historically, the reception area of the office has been the most neglected and underrated. Too often in physical therapy practices, a few chairs and magazines are considered sufficient for the waiting room. This area has become increasingly more important. It provides the client's first visual impression. It makes a definite statement regarding the practice, so that the patient will have certain expectations. Setting a positive climate by an attractively furnished reception area provides the right image and enhances promotional efforts.

WAITING ROOM CHECKLIST

Atmosphere appropriate to the practice	____	Easy access through doors	____
Adequate size (15 to 20 square feet per person)	____	Reading light	____
		Buzzer upon arrival	____
Magazine rack with current magazines	____	Easy and close access to bathroom	____
Coat and umbrella stand	____	Children's area (optional)	____
Patient pleasers (e.g., aquarium, plants, music)	____	Visibility of business office	____
Sufficient seating	____	Comfortable place to fill out insurance forms	____
Comfortable and therapeutic seating	____	Phone (optional)	____
		VCR/TV (optional)	____

Treatment Rooms

Personal preference and projected patient population will determine whether treatment rooms will be curtained or enclosed by walls. There are advantages to both arrangements. Curtained treatment rooms or cubicles provide greater flexibility; facilitate movement of therapy equipment from one cubicle to the next; are cheaper to construct; and provide for greater interaction between patients from cubicle to cubicle. Individual treatment rooms constructed with walls afford greater privacy, a more polished look, the ability to change the intended use, and better climate control.

TREATMENT ROOM CHECKLIST

Individual light switches	_____	Stool	_____
		Doorway strategically placed for privacy	_____
Adequate space for bilateral access to treatment table (at least 30 inches on each side)	_____		
		Sink (optional)	_____
		Proximity to other treatment rooms	_____
Clothing hooks with shelf below	_____		
		Outlets for equipment 36 inches above floor toward head of table	_____
Mirror (optional)	_____		
Chair with armrest	_____		

Hydrotherapy Room

Projected patient volume, referral sources, and intended services will determine whether a stationary whirlpool bath should be installed. Whirlpool installation is a major expense and source of trouble. Other alternatives include using a portable whirlpool that requires no special plumbing hookups, using an inexpensive noncommercial home model for hands or feet, or not providing the service at all. If a stationary whirlpool is going to be installed, the practitioner should be sure to obtain the manufacturer's templates, find a plumber who has installed a whirlpool before, supply pictures of installed whirlpools to the plumber, and meticulously check over the blueprints and the rough-ins. This will prevent major problems.

HYDROTHERAPY ROOM CHECKLIST

Sufficient size for bilateral access to whirlpool with wheelchair or whirlpool chair	_____	Sink for washing hands	_____
		Paper towel and soap dispensers	_____
		Isolation capabilities	_____
Storage for dressing supplies	_____	Proper ventilation	_____
		Canted floor drain	_____

HYDROTHERAPY ROOM CHECKLIST *continued*

Hot and cold water valves for hose next to whirlpool to be used for cleaning whirlpool and floor _____

Plumbing hookups for whirlpool installation according to manufacturer's template _____

Ceramic tile, water-resistant paint, or wall covering around the whirlpool _____

Phone jack (optional) _____

Exercise/Gymnasium Fitness Area

Personal preference, treatment philosophy, patient population, and projected services will determine whether a large room will be dedicated to exercise. This room can include mat tables, isokinetic equipment, dedicated weight machines, stationary bicycles, treadmills, and whatever other equipment will enhance the practice. An area such as this promotes patient interaction, increases therapist efficiency, and has excellent promotional value for distinguishing a physical therapy practice from a chiropractic office.

FITNESS AREA CHECKLIST

Adequate size for all major equipment _____

Dedicated line for isokinetic equipment _____

Mirrors on a portion of the walls _____

Reinforced walls for wall-mounted equipment _____

Water cooler _____

Durable floor covering _____

Additional Rooms

PATIENT BATHROOM CHECKLIST

Raised toilet or adapter _____

Wheelchair accessibility _____

Clothing hooks _____

Mirror _____

PATIENT BATHROOM CHECKLIST *continued*

Sink   _____   Proximity to treatment   _____
                                               rooms
Handrails   _____

STORAGE CHECKLIST

Generous space for   _____   Strategic location   _____
patient records, linen
(towels, sheets,   Ergonomic viability   _____
pillowcases, patient
gowns), medical
supplies, office supplies,
small equipment,
garbage awaiting
removal, water bottles
and cups for cooler,
cleaning supplies, and
coffee supplies

LAUNDRY/UTILITY ROOM CHECKLIST

Special electrical outlets   _____   Hot water heater   _____
for washer and dryer   (optional)

Vent for dryer   _____   Room for
                                               mop storage   _____
Water hookup   _____

BUSINESS OFFICE CHECKLIST

Visibility of front door   _____   Auditory privacy   _____
and reception area
Adequate size (100 feet   _____   Storage space for   _____
per person)   everyday supplies

BUSINESS OFFICE CHECKLIST *continued*

Sufficient counter space   _____   Phone access   _____
(18- to 24-inch depth)
                                             Outlet access   _____
Accessibility of files   _____
                                             Garbage pails   _____
Traffic flow control   _____
point for entering and   Storage for copier and   _____
exiting patients   supplies

PRIVATE OFFICE CHECKLIST

Adequate size   _____

Appropriate seating   _____
arrangement

Privacy from waiting   _____
room

Creation of desired   _____
image

PROFESSIONAL STAFF OFFICE CHECKLIST

Adequate size for   _____   Visibility of major   _____
projected number of   treatment area
professional staff
                                             Privacy for discussing   _____
Telephone jacks and   _____   patients
outlets strategically
placed   Shelves, uniform hooks,   _____
                                             and adequate storage

CONSTRUCTION PHASE

It would be futile to mention all the possible mishaps that can befall the
practitioner during construction. The practitioner's total dedication and patience
will be tested throughout this final phase of the project. Regardless of the con-

tractor, the practitioner should spend substantial time on site during construction. This will guarantee catching mistakes before they happen and being able to make last minute changes and to ensure that the promised materials are being used. It will also minimize mistakes and far-fetched interpretations of the final blueprint.

The construction industry sets acceptable deviation standards, which can create havoc with the design. For example, when a floor drain has been placed in the hydrotherapy room, the floor is expected to be level and not graded uphill. However, the industry allows a set deviation from level surface that will leave water in corners rather than in the drain.

Constant vigilance is the only way to prevent errors during construction. Certain manners must be observed so that the practitioner does not assume an adversarial role toward the construction workers. If the architect is overseeing the project, all major complaints or suggestions should be brought to the architect; otherwise, requests and questions should be brought to the general contractor or the contractor's designated superintendent. Interrupting the workers with questions and concerns disrupts their work. Major inspections and measurements should be done during construction breaks or off-hours.

Any changes requested by the tenant that are not on the final blueprint are generally made at the tenant's expense. The practitioner should be decisive and try to minimize changes that are not critical to the design.

Foundation

Foundation construction is necessary only if the office suite is located in a one-story building. One-story buildings generally have a concrete slab as the subfloor, and the floor covering goes directly on top of the concrete slab. If this is the case, all the plumbing, utility lines, and floor drains must be installed before pouring the concrete slab.

If the slab has already been poured before the lease is signed, it will have to be chopped up in those areas where plumbing and utility lines are relocated. If a stationary whirlpool is included in the plans, it is recommended that a floor drain be installed and canted so that water will run into the drain. Chopping up the floor is an extremely noisy and dusty procedure. Once the work has been completed, cement will be poured to patch up the floor, which must then be inspected to make sure that it is finished smoothly and leveled.

Framing

The partitions or skeleton walls are created by using 2 by 4 inch studs, which may be either wood or metal depending on the building code. This phase is completed very quickly, but the speed can be very misleading because the illusion is created that if everything else goes as quickly, the office suite will be completed 2 months ahead of schedule.

Once the studs are installed, a three-dimensional visualization of the plan on the blueprint is available by standing in the office suite. Practitioners should spend an evening or weekend "living" in the suite and walking through typical routines in the workday. This will provide a feel for the adequacy of the individual dimensions. Once the sheetrock and doors are installed, the dimensions of each room will be decreased by approximately 2 to 3 inches. It is in the best interest of the practitioner to check the dimensions of every room, hallway, closet, and window against the blueprint. It is not uncommon to find errors by the carpenters. Moreover, the practitioner might have a change of heart once the dimensions of a particular room are visualized clearly. In either case the contractor must be notified before the next phase of construction.

FRAMING CHECKLIST

Door frames	_____	Wall reinforcement as indicated on blueprint	_____
Closets	_____		
Individual rooms	_____	Studs 16 inches apart, as per code	_____

Rough-Ins

Once the skeleton walls or studs are up, the plumbers, electricians, and any other workers needed for installations within the walls arrive on the scene. They work simultaneously, installing ducts, tubing, pipes, and conduits for all systems and utilities. All the lines installed within the walls are attached to the main hookups running through the ceiling.

Once again, meticulous inspection of the placement of all installations is required. The practitioner must remember that the construction industry allows a set deviation in distance from that specified on the blueprint and beware accordingly. All the equipment manufacturer's templates should be used to ensure accurate placement of electrical lines around the major equipment. Special attention to plumbing lines is required if stationary whirlpools are being installed.

Additional information is available from the plumbing and electrical checklists in this chapter.

Inspections

When the rough-ins are completed, the local building inspectors arrive to confirm that the work was performed as designated on the blueprint. The next phase can not be initiated without the approval of the inspectors. The individual inspections lead to the granting of the certificate of occupancy, which is necessary before the doors can be opened to patients.

Walls

Before placement of the sheetrock or wallboards, any soundproofing and insulation materials must be installed. The sheetrock is installed by the carpenters with nails. The nails leave holes, and the sheetrock leaves uneven seams. Once all the sheetrock is in place, a spackler arrives to spackle and tape. This is a process whereby a spackling compound is applied over all holes and ridges to create a smooth surface. The seams are generally handled with special taping material, which is then sanded down to provide a smooth surface. The purpose of both procedures is to provide a smooth, durable surface for painting or wallpapering.

The final step in preparing the walls is priming and sealing by the painter, to be followed by painting or installation of wallpaper. Painting can be done by rolling, brush strokes, or spraying. The latter method should be used with caution; it is a faster technique but is messy and leaves inconsistencies in color and texture if done incorrectly.

If the blueprint calls for a dropped ceiling which seems to be the industry norm, the framing for the ceiling tiles will be installed concurrently with the wall preparation.

WALL CONSTRUCTION CHECKLIST

Smooth walls and corners	_____	Leftover paint saved for future use	_____
Paint confined to walls	_____	Level ceiling line	_____
Paint applied evenly without shadows or drips	_____	Tiles even in frames	_____
		No defective tiles	_____

Finishing

The finishing phase includes installation of ceiling tiles, hardware, switch and outlet covers, and baseboards; staining of doors; and a host of other minor touches to give a visibly finished environment. It is tedious, time-consuming work, which frequently is not done to the tenant's satisfaction. Most of the problems during this stage are easily rectified.

Punch List

When the construction workers have cleaned up the site and removed all unused construction materials, the tenant must compile a *punch list*, which is a list of all the work not completed to the tenant's satisfaction. It will take many walks through the office to compile a comprehensive list. When the list is complete, the tenant should make an appointment with the landlord's representative and the general contractor to walk through the office together. This will give the practitioner the opportunity to discuss the deficiencies. The contractor will then call back a few workers to address the agreed-upon problems. This process continues for quite a while until all items on the list have been satisfactorily corrected.

INTERIOR DESIGN ITEMS

Interior decorating commences on the day the lease is signed. It includes the selection of wall coverings, floor coverings, window treatments, patient furniture, office furniture, and built-in cabinets. If the decision has been made to hire an interior decorator, these selections and the entire process will be coordinated by the decorator.

If an interior decorator has not been hired, the private practitioner must start the process immediately upon signing the lease. Everything agreed upon between any of the providers and the practitioner must be confirmed in writing. Manufacturer's product numbers, pictures, and samples of agreed-upon materials and products should be kept in a file by the practitioner in case of potential conflicts.

Built-In Cabinets

The first step is to decide whether built-in cabinets are essential to the design of the office suite. Built-ins are likely to be a major expense and to take a long time to build, and they can not be reinstalled if the office suite does not work out. The advantages of built-ins are that they provide maximum efficiency in utilizing available space, confer an extremely professional look, and are customized to the unique needs of the practice.

The three major sources of cabinets are local furniture cabinetmakers, kitchen cabinetmakers, and major cabinet manufacturing companies. In deciding which of these to use, account must be taken of the cabinetmaker's reputation before considering the price estimate quoted by each. References should definitely be checked and previous work inspected. Questions to be asked of previous customers are as follows:

1. Were the cabinets delivered and installed on time?
2. Was the price competitive?
3. Was the installation handled professionally, leaving no damage to the existing space?
4. Are the cabinets holding up, without loosening of hardware or changes in fit?
5. Did the company and all its personnel handle themselves professionally and live up to their contractual agreement?

Patient and Office Furniture

The earlier furniture is ordered, the more likely its delivery will coincide with the projected opening day. Its selection is based on the intended image of the office, budgetary constraints, for whose use the furniture is intended, and how long the furniture is expected to last.

There are many sources of furniture. If the budget and expected volume of the practice demand use of contract furniture, this must be ordered from office or commercial furniture suppliers. Contract furniture is furniture specifically designed and manufactured for commercial use. It is more durable than residential furniture, is generally more expensive, and has previously been known for its more austere look, although recently aesthetic considerations have been included in its design.

If the budget does not allow for the purchase of contract furniture, there are many other sources. Chairs, tables, sofas, lamps, and other items can be ordered from residential furniture suppliers. Fabrics can be custom-ordered, or items can be purchased from stock.

If ample time is available the practitioner should consider ordering directly from furniture manufacturers. Most companies are located in the southeast region of the United States, and telephone numbers can be obtained from decorating magazines. This may save approximately one-third of the purchase price. The disadvantages of dealing over the phone with these companies is that the order is placed without seeing the furniture, and the projected delivery time is usually longer than when ordering from local furniture stores.

Floor Covering

Flooring provides the largest expanse of color in the office except for the walls. It should be sturdy enough to handle anticipated traffic as well as the weight of the equipment that moves over it. It should have low maintenance requirements, match the decor of the office, and be safe for the patients. The most frequently used flooring materials are carpeting, vinyl sheeting, ceramic tiles, and linoleum tiles.

FLOOR COVERING CHECKLIST

Low maintenance requirements	_____	Durable	_____
		Stain-resistant	_____
Easy and safe to move on	_____	Aesthetically pleasing and consistent with image	_____
Sound-absorbent	_____		

SUMMARY

Office planning and design can be a fulfilling experience, but it should be approached cautiously and methodically. This chapter has provided information and organizational guidelines to enable the practitioner to design an efficient and pleasing office suite.

SUGGESTED READINGS

Cotton H: You can't do work with poor tools. p. 59. In Medical Practice Management. Medical Economics Books, Oradell, NJ, 1985

Johnston BE, Lord PJ: Planning and developing the facility. p. 129. In Your Private Practice. Vol. 2. Planning and Organization. Peter J. Lord & Associates, Lake City, FL, 1982

Magistro CM: Department planning, design, and construction. p. 59. In Hickok RJ (ed): Physical Therapy Administration and Management. Williams & Wilkins, Baltimore, 1981

Malkin J: The Design of Medical and Dental Facilities. Van Nostrand Reinhold, New York, 1981

Schwartz M: Designing and Building Your Own Professional Office. Medical Economics Books, Oradell, NJ, 1982

Schwartz M: Remodeling Your Professional Office. Medical Economics Books, Oradell, NJ, 1985

7

POLICIES AND PROCEDURES

Many businesses do not provide written guidelines and methods for employees to follow. However, in the health care field, where the persons served are not just clients but also patients, strict protocols must be used to ensure patient safety and well-being. Strict procedure must be followed for infection control and the correct technique used for procedures such as ultrasound treatments, electrical stimulation, and whirlpool baths. A manual that details in writing these policies and procedures should be kept in every facility and be readily accessible to employees. The manual acts as a handy reference guide and a good teaching tool, and it details the specific operational policies and procedures that the practice wants to enforce. Many regulatory authorities, accrediting agencies, insurance companies, and health insurance organizations, as well as Medicare require the private practice to have a policy and procedure manual on the premises.

Each facility writes its own policy and procedure manual because the manual must be specific for the individual practice. Clinical, environmental and safety, and pertinent administrative policies and procedures are essential for the private practice, but it is desirable also to include financial and personnel protocols in the manual. Some regulatory authorities even mandate which policies and procedures are required for a facility; however, they do not mandate the wording, format, or style, which are all decided by the owners of the facility.

Many people may be familiar with policies and procedures of their business when these are provided in the form of handbooks, of which the most common type is the employee handbook. This usually describes in detail the company's personnel policies and procedures and may include topics such as employee benefits and disciplinary procedures for absenteeism.

Before writing a policy and procedure manual, it is necessary to define the subject area covered (e.g., authorization for continuing education and expenses). A *policy* sets guidelines for the standard operation of the private practice; therefore the term standard operating policies (SOPs) is often used. A *procedure* is the method by which a policy will be implemented. Policies and procedures must always be written in the format that the facility has chosen. Verbal policies and procedures are unacceptable, as are memoranda and interoffice communications. Policies can be written without procedures if appropriate.

It is the responsibility of the facility adminstrator or head therapist to disseminate the information in the policy and procedure manual to the entire staff. The information should be presented during employee orientation and updated or reinforced at regular intervals at staff meetings. Many accrediting agencies and regulatory authorities require that each policy and procedure be reviewed and necessary revisions made annually. Policies and procedures that have been revised must be kept on file in their original as well as updated form to provide proof that they have been updated. A good rule of thumb is to save all formal paperwork for 7 years. Each policy and procedure must show the date of revision, and a cover page should be placed at the beginning of each manual showing yearly approval of the manual along with the facility administrator's signature. A copy of the policy and procedure manual(s) should be kept in the administrative area and the staff office. The business office should also have its own copy if it is located in a separate area, as should any other separate department. If the practice has several departments, it may be appropriate to write not only a policy and procedure manual for the entire facility but one for each separate department as well. The contents of the different manuals need not overlap except where the same policies and procedures apply to more than one department.

REGULATORY AUTHORITIES

The policies and procedures must be in full compliance with the requirements of all authorities that regulate the practice, including the state licensing agency under whose jurisdiction it falls. All applicable local, state, and federal authorities must be contacted to ensure that no agency has been omitted. Occupational permits or licenses from the town, city, and county may also be required. If the practice plans to obtain Medicare certification, it must set policies and procedures that adhere to Health Care Financing Administration (HCFA) rules and regulations. A copy of these rules and regulations can be obtained from the state office of licensure and certification.

The current HCFA regulations pertinent to the private practice are part of regulations No. 5, subpart Q. These regulations are numbered 405.1730 through 405.1737 and are entitled "Conditions for Coverage: Outpatient Physical Therapy Services Furnished by Physical Therapists in Independent Practice" (HCFA, 405.1730 to 405.1737); regulation 405.232(e) also pertains to outpatient physical therapy procedures and must be adhered to. Since these Medicare policies and procedures are so important to many private practitioners, an example of a policy and procedure for regulations 405.1731 to 405.1736 is provided in Appendix 7-2 at the end of the chapter. However, these policies and procedures and those for regulation 405.1737 must be written so that they are appropriate for the particular practice. Much of the language can be and has been taken directly from the regulations, since these set the requirements that must be followed.

Certification as a rehabilitation agency demands adherence to certain rules. The above policies and procedures may need to be expanded or even changed. Information on the requirements for this certification can be obtained from the state office of licensure and certification.

Fire and safety issues as required by the local fire marshal should also be addressed. The fire marshal should be contacted several months before the facility's opening to ensure that the facility complies with the local rules.

Accreditation from the Commission for the Accreditation for Rehabilitation Facilities (CARF) for outpatient services or for outpatient services and a specialty program require even more policies and procedures. The CARF standards can be obtained by writing to CARF, 500 North Pantano Road, Tucson, AZ 85715.

Facilities not only must be careful that the policies they have written for a particular agency or regulatory authority are in compliance but they must also make certain that these policies are not contradicted by any other policy and procedure in the manual. Clinical policies and procedures must also be described in a clinically correct manner and must be carried out in the way they are written. For example, if the private practice's administrator has written a detailed policy and procedure stating that a certain additive is to be put into the whirlpool bath before every whirlpool treatment, that particular additive must be used or the policy and procedure must be changed to provide a generic description, to specify a different additive, or to allow various additives. If an inspector finds an additive being used that is not provided for in the policy and procedure manual, the facility may be cited for not following its own policies and procedures. The facility administrator may choose to be either very general or very specific in writing policies and procedures. For example, for ultrasound treatment a general policy and procedure is usually acceptable, but the administrator may want to have a specific ultrasound procedure for each particular brand and model of equipment.

TYPES OF POLICIES AND PROCEDURES

For a private practice, five types of policies and procedures will be discussed:

1. Administrative
2. Personnel
3. Financial
4. Environmental and safety
5. Clinical

Administrative

Administrative policies and procedures focus on the general operation of the practice, including:

Purpose and function of the practice
Description of services
Hours of operation

Supervision of services
Coordination of services with those provided by other organizations or in-
    dividuals
Referrals
Physician's directions
Plan of care
Abbreviations
Physical therapy records
Exchange of physical therapy records and reports
Release of physical therapy records
Standards of documentation

Personnel

Personnel policies and procedures relate to the human resources of the facility.
Any information that the employees need about benefits or organizational structure or about what is expected of them during the workday (from work standards
to dress code) should be included in this section. Examples of personnel policies
and procedures may include

Organizational structure
Professional standards
Employment procedures
Nondiscrimination
Orientation program
Workers' compensation
Benefits
Resignations
Disciplinary action
Education reimbursement
Dress code
Job descriptions

There are many federal and state laws that dictate rules regarding employees.
The facility administrator or personnel director should be familiar with these
laws so that all personnel policies can comply with and not contradict government regulations. These regulations include overtime rules for nonsalaried workers and right-to-work laws within particular states.

Financial

Financial policies and procedures are important so that all employees may
realize that they have an obligation to promote the financial well-being of the
organization. The financial policies and procedures also give guidelines for budgetary planning, inventory control, writing off bad debts, and requesting reimbursement checks. The business office staff should be able to refer to the manual

on a regular basis to obtain information on how to perform routine functions. Policies and procedures that may be included in this section are

Budget preparation
Inventory control
Purchasing
Capital equipment
Request for reimbursement checks
Petty cash funds
Credit and collections
Indigent patients
Insurance billing
Travel and education requests
Travel allowance
Expense reports

Environmental and Safety

The environmental and safety section covers those policies and procedures affecting the plant itself, life safety measures, infection control, control of hazardous wastes (if on premises), and maintenance practices for the building and equipment. Among the pertinent policies and procedures for the organization may be

Emergency medical procedures
Fire and safety plan
Cleaning procedures
Infection control
Disposal of contaminated wastes
Maintenance plan
Smoking policy
Risk management

Clinical

Clinical policies and procedures should exist for the operation of each piece of equipment and for routine clinical procedures or programs. Indications and contraindications need to be listed where appropriate. Examples of items covered by clinical policies and procedures include

Whirlpool
Isokinetic testing and training equipment
High-voltage galvanic stimulator
Interferential therapy
Ultrasound
Paraffin

Hot pack machine
Cold pack machine
Intermittent compression pump
Burn and open wound protocol
Therapeutic exercise techniques
Treadmill
Exercise bicycle
Biofeedback
Weight lifting equipment
Direct-current stimulator
Iontophoresis
Transcutaneous electrical nerve stimulator
Functional electrical stimulator
Back protocol
Arthritis program
Evaluation forms

This section can be quite extensive depending on the size of the practice, the number of specialty programs available, whether or not support personnel are allowed to assist with treatment, and the amount and type of equipment owned. If support personnel are used, a policy must exist for an orientation and training program that allows the supervising person to check off competencies as they are achieved.

CONTENT OF POLICIES AND PROCEDURES

Each policy and procedure should include at a minimum the following:

1. *Subject:* the topic; what the policy and procedure is about (e.g., whirlpools)
2. *Standard operating procedure (SOP) number:* the number assigned to the particular policy and procedure (see section below on SOP numbers for a more detailed explanation)
3. *Effective date:* the date the policy goes into effect
4. *Type of policy:* administrative, personnel, financial, environmental and safety, or clinical
5. *Date reviewed with approval signature:* reviewed initially and yearly thereafter; signed by the private practice's administrator and sometimes by the president of the board of directors, if applicable
6. *Policy:* guideline to the practice's operation
7. *Procedure:* method to achieve policy

Many facilities also include purpose, scope, and responsibility in the format of their policies. *Purpose* states the reason why the policy is being written. *Scope* relates to whom the policy affects (e.g., clinical versus clerical staff). *Responsibility* defines who has the supervisory accountability for carrying out the policy and procedure. Use of these additional categories can help clarify discrepancies that may arise as practices grow larger and the number of employees and the chance for confusion increase.

SOP NUMBERS

Standard operating policies are usually numbered according to the subject area that they cover. Since five major categories of policies and procedures have been used, they will be labeled as such:

Administrative	1.000
Personnel	2.000
Financial	3.000
Environmental and safety	4.000
Clinical	5.000

An administrative policy and procedure entitled Purpose and Function of the Practice would be numbered 1.001 if it were the first policy in that section, 1.015 if it were the fifteenth, and so on. A clinical policy on ultrasound would be numbered 5.005 if it were the fifth policy in that section. Any numbering system that will work well for the practice can be used.

POLICY AND PROCEDURE CHECKLIST

Policy   _____

Procedure   _____

Contents of the policy   _____
and procedure format

Five types of policies   _____
and procedures used

Four examples of   _____
administrative policies
and procedures

Four examples of   _____
financial policies and
procedures

SUGGESTED READINGS

Lord PJ, Johnston BE Jr: Your Private Practice. Administration. Practice Dynamics, Lake City, FL, 1983

U.S. Health Care Financing Administration: Medicare Regulations No. 5, Subpart Q, 405.1730 to 405.1737 and 405.232(e). 44.7–76.

APPENDIX 7-1

SAMPLE FORMAT

Sample format for a policy and procedure is demonstrated below.

PHYSICAL THERAPY COMPANY X

S.O.P. NUMBER _____

TYPE OF POLICY _____

EFFECTIVE DATE _____

SUBJECT: _____

POLICY: _____

PROCEDURE: _____

DATE REVIEWED _____

APPROVAL SIGNATURE _____ TITLE _____

APPENDIX 7-2

EXAMPLES OF POLICIES AND PROCEDURES

The following policies and procedures have been written to demonstrate an example of what was required to receive Medicare certification according to regulations 405.1730 to 405.1736 in 1988.

PHYSICAL THERAPY COMPANY X

S.O.P. NUMBER	1.011
TYPE OF POLICY	ADMINISTRATIVE
EFFECTIVE DATE	JANUARY 1, 19--

SUBJECT: LICENSURE AND SUPERVISION OF PERSONNEL

POLICY: All physical therapists must be currently licensed in the state or hold a temporary permit. Any therapist holding a temporary permit will be supervised by a physical therapist holding a current license. There must be a licensed physical therapist on the premises whenever physical therapy services are rendered in the facility. In Physical Therapy Company X's practice, all physical therapy services will be rendered on the premises.

PROCEDURE: Proof of licensure is required by evidence of a current license, which is to be displayed in the waiting room. Therapists with a temporary permit must bring in the temporary permit, which is also to be hung in the waiting room. Verification that the licensee is in good standing with the state will be done by the administrator by phone call before the employment of the therapist.

A currently licensed physical therapist must be on the premises whenever patient services are rendered. Scheduling of the licensed physical therapists will be done by the administrator.

DATE REVIEWED _____

APPROVAL SIGNATURE _____ TITLE _____

PHYSICAL THERAPY COMPANY X

S.O.P. NUMBER   1.012

TYPE OF POLICY   ADMINISTRATIVE

EFFECTIVE DATE   JANUARY 1, 19--

SUBJECT: PHYSICIAN'S DIRECTION AND PLAN OF CARE

POLICY: Services rendered to patients must be only on the order of a physician who has indicated the anticipated goals of the patient and who is responsible for the general medical direction of such services as part of the total care of the patient. There must be a written plan of care for each patient, which is reviewed every thirty days by the patient's physician. Pertinent medical information must be made available to the physical therapist before or at the start of treatment.

PROCEDURE: 1.   Before or at the start of therapy services, the physical therapist must be aware of the following:
  a.   The patient's significant past history
  b.   Diagnosis(es)
  c.   Physician's orders
  d.   Rehabilitation goals and potential for their achievement
  e.   Contraindications, if any
  f.   The extent to which the patient is aware of the diagnosis and prognosis
  g.   Where appropriate, the summary of treatment rendered and results achieved during previous periods of physical therapy services or institutionalization

2.   There is a written plan of care, established by the physician, which indicates anticipated goals and specifies the type, amount, frequency, and duration of physical therapy services. Where appropriate, the plan is developed in consultation between the physical therapist and the patient's attending physician. The plan of care and results of treatment are reviewed once every thirty days, or more if required, by the attending physician and the physical therapist, and the indicated action is taken.

3.   Patients are seen by a physician at least once every thirty days. General medical direction at appropriate intervals is evidenced from the clinical record.

4.   The attending physician is promptly notified of any changes in the patient's condition. If changes are required in the plan of care, such changes are approved by the attending physician and noted in the clinical record.

(Adapted into a policy and procedure from Medicare Regulations No. 5, Subpart Q, 405.1733)

DATE REVIEWED _____
APPROVAL SIGNATURE _____   TITLE _____

PHYSICAL THERAPY COMPANY X

S.O.P. NUMBER	1.013
TYPE OF POLICY	ADMINISTRATIVE
EFFECTIVE DATE	JANUARY 1, 19—

SUBJECT: PHYSICAL THERAPY SERVICES

POLICY: A quality program of physical therapy services with state of the art equipment is available for patients.

PROCEDURE: Physical therapy services utilizing therapeutic exercise and the modalities of heat, cold, water, and electricity will be provided. An evaluation is to be conducted on every patient that includes tests and measurements of strength, balance, endurance, range of motion, and activities of daily living. These services are provided by a licensed physical therapist.

(Adapted into a policy and procedure from Medicare Regulations No. 5, Subpart Q, 405.1734)

DATE REVIEWED _____

APPROVAL SIGNATURE _____ TITLE _____

PHYSICAL THERAPY COMPANY X

S.O.P. NUMBER	1.014
TYPE OF POLICY	ADMINISTRATIVE
EFFECTIVE DATE	JANUARY 1, 19—

SUBJECT: COORDINATION OF SERVICES WITH OTHER ORGANIZA-TIONS, AGENCIES, OR INDIVIDUALS

POLICY: The physical therapy services provided by the physical therapist in independent practice are coordinated with health and medical services provided to the patients by organizations, agencies, or individuals.

PROCEDURE: When a patient is receiving or has recently received health and medical services from providers, organizations, physicians, or others that are related to and may involve the physical therapy program, the physical therapist shall, on a regular basis, exchange with such providers, organizations, physicians, or others, in accordance with the policy on clinical records, documented information that has a bearing on the patient health and welfare so as to ensure that services effectively complement one another.

(Adapted into a policy and procedure from Medicare Regulations No. 5, Subpart Q, 405.1735)

DATE REVIEWED _____

APPROVAL SIGNATURE _____ TITLE _____

PHYSICAL THERAPY COMPANY X

S.O.P. NUMBER   1.015

TYPE OF POLICY   ADMINISTRATIVE

EFFECTIVE DATE   JANUARY 1, 19--

SUBJECT: CLINICAL RECORDS

POLICY: The physical therapist maintains clinical records on all patients in accordance with accepted professional standards and practices. The clinical records are completely and accurately documented, readily accessible, and systematically organized to facilitate retrieving and compiling information.

PROCEDURE: 1. Clinical record information is recognized as confidential and is stored in a fire-proof, locked cabinet in the business office.
2. A patient's written consent is required for release of information not authorized by law.
3. The clinical record will contain sufficient information to identify the patient clearly, to justify the diagnosis(es) and treatment, and to document the results accurately. All clinical records must contain the following general categories of data:
   A. Documented evidence of the assessment of the needs of the patient, of an appropriate plan of care, and of the care and services provided
   B. Identification data and consent forms
   C. Medical history
   D. Report of physical examinations(s), if any
   E. Observations and progress notes
   F. Reports of treatments and clinical findings
   G. Discharge summary including final diagnosis(es) and prognosis
4. Current clinical records and those of discharged patients are completed promptly.
5. All clinical information pertaining to a patient is centralized in the patient's clinical record.
6. Clinical records are retained for a period of seven years, or more if required by state statute.
7. Clinical records are indexed according to the name of the patient (last name first, then first name, then middle initial) to facilitate acquisition of statistical clinical information and retrieval of records for administrative action.

(Adapted into a policy and procedure from Medicare Regulations No. 5, Subpart Q, 405.1735).

DATE REVIEWED _____
APPROVAL SIGNATURE _____   TITLE _____

PHYSICAL THERAPY COMPANY X

S.O.P. NUMBER   1.016

TYPE OF POLICY   ADMINISTRATIVE

EFFECTIVE DATE   JANUARY 1, 19--

SUBJECT: RELEASE OF MEDICAL RECORDS

POLICY: Medical records will be released only with the patient's written consent for release of medical records, or by court order.

PROCEDURE: 1.   The patient must sign a Release of Information form. In the case of a minor, the parent or legal guardian must sign the Release of Information form. This form will be kept in the patient's clinical record.
2.   No original records will be released from the facility except by court order. Copies will be made for the patients at a charge of ten cents per page.

DATE REVIEWED _____

APPROVAL SIGNATURE _____   TITLE _____

8

STAFFING

The greatest monthly operating expense for a private physical therapy practice is that for the staff. Staff persons provide all the services, including clinical care of patients and all related administrative activities necessary to run the office and collect payments. Therefore, staffing requirements must be considered for two separate units: the professional staff, which provides patient care and performs related functions, and the administrative staff, which is responsible for administrative and clerical functions.

Many professional and administrative services must be performed for a private physical therapy practice to be successful. Moreover, staff members may be responsible for one or for many activities, depending upon the number of employees and the practice's business volume. Therefore, this chapter will discuss staff functions rather than the titles of the persons performing them. Each private practice can decide how to group activities under job categories and assign them to specific employees.

PROFESSIONAL ACTIVITIES

Patient Care

The most important activity provided by the professional staff is patient care, which is the actual provision of physical therapy services to patients. Depending upon the philosophy of the private practice, various modes of delivering these services are available.

Where there is considerable hands-on therapy, physical therapists and physical therapist assistants will provide most of the treatment. Where there is considerable use of machines, physical therapist assistants and in some instances aides may provide most of the treatment. The philosophy and goals of the private practice determine what level of personnel will provide patient care (see Ch. 1).

The private practitioner must always remember that high-quality patient care is the primary service to be provided. Therefore, selection of the physical therapy clinicians may prove critical for the growth and development of the private practice.

Equipment Purchases and Repairs

At least one of the physical therapists on the staff should be responsible for the equipment, all of which must be in working order for patient safety. Furthermore, physical therapy equipment is rapidly and constantly changing, and therefore someone in the practice must keep abreast of new equipment developments. It is a common practice for local vendors to lend equipment to physical therapy practices in the hope of an eventual sale. Use of borrowed equipment enables the private practice to keep up with the new technology, which is also helpful when purchasing equipment.

Inventory and Supply Purchases

At least one of the staff physical therapists should be responsible for maintaining the inventory of professional supplies (e.g., biofeedback electrodes, ultrasound gel, and lightweight corsets), since they are used constantly. There is no more frustrating feeling then being unable to provide the quality care chosen because the necessary supplies are lacking. When a specific supply item runs low, additional supplies should be ordered. This task of inventory and supply purchase is time-consuming, as supply volume can change rapidly. It becomes even more time-consuming if the private practice elects to sell professional supplies to patients.

Written Correspondence

The written correspondence required of the professional staff will vary among individual private practices. Daily entries on the patients' charts, letters to referring physicians, and responses to attorneys are but three of the time-consuming written tasks. Dictation may save the professionals some time but requires transcription by the administrative staff. In many private practices the timing of written correspondence becomes a critical issue. For example, if a progress report is to be hand carried by a patient to the physician, this report is given priority. Written correspondence is a very time-consuming job requirement for the professional staff and time must be allocated properly.

Public Relations

Public relations is a 24-hour per day task for the private practice and its staff. Private practitioners must remember that at any given moment they may meet a prospective referral source or patient. Therefore they must always present themselves to the public in an appropriate light. In addition, physical therapists can provide excellent public relations by the manner in which they care for their patients; this may prove more important than the quality of care rendered. A patient is more likely to respond to a warm, considerate professional than to a rude, abrupt one. Simple consideration of the patient may create excellent public relations for the practice, for example, when physical therapists come to the waiting room to inform patients that they are slightly behind schedule. Patients respond favorably to considerate gestures. The practitioner should remember that patients almost always talk about their health providers to their friends. If the patients speak highly of the practice, the reputation of the practice will be enhanced.

Marketing/Promotion

The physical therapy private practice must continually carry on the marketing phase of the business. It may prove helpful to have one of the professional staff be responsible for promotional activities, thereby allowing for coordination among all employees and for an organized and systematic approach to marketing the private practice (see Ch. 10).

Continuing Education

Continuing education is one method of keeping the professional staff up to date with changes in physical therapy. It may prove helpful for one member of the professional staff to coordinate continuing education by screening courses, allowing employees time off to attend courses, and scheduling patient coverage.

In-Service Education

In-service education is a method by which the professional staff can educate themselves and each other. Meetings may be scheduled on a weekly, monthly, or semimonthly basis at which different professionals can present the new information that they obtained in continuing education courses and outside speakers can instruct the professional staff on new developments. Once again, it may prove most efficient for one person to coordinate the program.

Meetings

Meetings among the professional staff can be held weekly or as needed. Such meetings permit people with similar responsibilities to communicate, help in maintaining consistency among the individual practitioners, and allow the professional staff to critique and alter present policies. Allowing the professional staff members to have input into policies and procedures facilitates compliance (see Ch. 7).

Professional Activities

Professionals should be involved in professional activities either in their national and state professional associations or in their local communities. Coordination of such activities for a large professional staff is very time consuming, but professionally related activities give the physical therapy private practice valuable exposure, which can only help to promote its interests.

Clinical Education

Physical therapy education programs are constantly looking for high-quality physical therapists to instruct their students in clinical practice. As a professional responsibility, physical therapy private practices should, if at all possible, provide clinical education for affiliating students. To provide a high-quality learning experience, one member of the professional staff must assume responsibility for organizing and coordinating the education program, although the program itself may include additional professionals.

ADMINISTRATIVE ACTIVITIES
Telephone Reception

The person answering the telephone is in an extremely critical position, as the handling of incoming calls can have a great impact on the way the private physical therapy practice is perceived. The telephone receptionist serves as a symbol of the practice. It is important to speak in a sympathetic and sensitive voice while maintaining an aura of professionalism; brusqueness or rudeness could cause the caller to hang up. The telephone reception person is responsible for keeping all lines of communications open but may seek assistance from other staff members if necessary. All telephone messages must be recorded on a dual copy pad so that one copy can be forwarded to the appropriate employee and another placed in a master book. Additionally, the telephone receptionist has to be as accommodating as possible to people who telephone the office. Appropriate behavior can promote solid public relations and thereby enhance the image of the private practice.

Office Reception

The job of office receptionist is a very difficult one, requiring a very friendly and sociable person to interact with the various patients and vendors who enter the office. All patients check in with the office receptionist, who informs the appropriate physical therapist that the patient has arrived. If this therapist happens to be behind schedule, it is the office receptionist with whom the patient is likely to become annoyed. A friendly office receptionist can set the tone for the patient's visit, and as previously stated, a patient who enjoys the therapy visits is valuable.

Chart Development

The development of a patient's chart is mandatory for all physical therapy practices. The patient must complete a personal information sheet, provide insurance information, and present the physician's referral. This information is placed in a folder, along with paper for the therapist to provide the appropriate documentation. Chart development also involves coding for easy retrieval and billing efficiency.

Mail

When the daily mail arrives, someone in the front office should sort it by placing it into piles for the appropriate employees. Checks should go to the person who posts the collections, invoices to the person who pays the bills, etc.

An active private practice receives all kinds of mail daily, including correspondence and bills for services rendered. In many offices the mail is delivered and picked up at the receptionist's window. If this practice is not followed, some other method of delivering and receiving mail must be instituted.

As part of the private practice's promotional efforts it will become necessary to mail information to many potential referral sources. This mass mailing should be the responsibility of one person and should be sent to all referral sources on the private practice's master list. The mailing task includes addressing envelopes, fliers, or brochures, stuffing envelopes if necessary, and placing the correct postage on the envelope. To economize on postage it may prove cost-effective to obtain a bulk mail permit from the post office.

Typing and Word Processing

In physical therapy private practice considerable correspondence must be carried on. This includes solicitations of new referral sources and frequent letters explaining the practice and thanking the referral sources for personal meetings. Correspondence about patient care is essential; since the practice of physical therapy depends primarily on referrals, physical therapists must keep the referring physicians abreast of each patient's progress. Communication with insurance companies and attorneys is necessary to receive payment for services rendered. The amount of typing or word processing required by a practice will increase proportionally as the practice grows.

Telephoning Patients

Patients frequently leave the office following a therapy session without making their next appointment or cancel appointments without rescheduling for another day. Failure to track patients who do not reschedule appointments frequently leads to lost patient visits, which in turn results in lost revenues and in some cases unhappy referral sources. The person in the office who handles patient follow-up should telephone patients who do not reschedule and ask them to make a new appointment.

Paying Bills

In the course of running a private physical therapy practice bills must be paid. The timeliness of payment is important for the credit and reputation of the practice. One person should be responsible for paying all bills. Bills should be paid according to an organized schedule. Two frequently used schedules are every second Friday or the fifteenth and the last day of every month.

Office Inventory and Supply Purchases

At least one member of the administrative staff should be responsible for office supplies, which are constantly being used and must be replenished. Stationery, envelopes, stamps, business cards, referral pads, brochures, and writing implements are but a few of the necessary office supplies. The owner of the practice may become very upset when needed supplies are not available. Lack of supplies can be a problem because of the time lag between ordering and receiving special order items, but with proper inventory procedures all items should always be readily available.

Dealing with Support People

Working with support people is time-consuming, and the time spent is not usually revenue-producing for the professional staff. Ideally, the administrative staff should work with the support people. For example, the job of deciding on and purchasing stationery items may be delegated to a member of the administrative staff, as may routine dealings with the accountant and attorney. Even the purchase of office equipment and supplies need not require the time and effort of the professional staff.

Office Cleaning

Most private practices have a cleaning service contract, either included in the office lease or negotiated separately. However, even with a cleaning service it is necessary to tidy up the office constantly, if not during the day then most definitely at the end of the day, so that the office will look presentable for the following day's early morning patients. While cleaning services clean, they do not straighten up the office by performing tasks such as placing the magazines and weights in the appropriate racks and changing linen.

Clothes Washing and Drying

An ongoing problem for a private physical therapy practice is linen, which includes sheets, pillowcases, towels, and patient gowns. The use of linen grows proportionally with the volume of the practice, and therefore, keeping it clean becomes a major problem. The cost of a linen service quickly becomes prohibitive for a growing practice, and a frequent solution is to purchase a clothes washer and dryer. The administrative staff usually becomes responsible for washing and drying the linen, which is very time-consuming as it includes folding the dried linen.

Posting the Patient's Treatment

Following every physical therapy session the charges must be posted to the patient's account. Posting means recording the charges in the patient's individual file and the clinic's master file, along with the appropriate International Classification of Diseases (ICD) procedure codes. The ICD procedure codes (contained in the ICD manual) are required by the insurance carriers. The posting can be done by the one-step entry method or can be handled by the computer if the office is computerized. Once the treatment session charges are posted, the billing process can begin.

Billing Patients and Insurance Companies

Billing patients and insurance companies is an administrative function that is crucial for survival of the practice. Bills should be mailed frequently. Private practitioners know that the longer a bill is outstanding after therapy, the more difficult it is to collect. Billing delays may occur when the administrative staff is overworked or the office is understaffed. Billing the patient following each therapy session is an excellent idea. If the practice has agreed to bill the insurance company, the patient must provide the correct information, which must be verified by the administrative staff. Furthermore, the smaller the bill, the faster the insurance company pays. If parties other than the patient or the insurance company (e.g., attorneys) are to be billed, the information should be verified. When billing an attorney in the event of an accident or a lawsuit, a medical lien, which secures payment from the attorney after the actual settlement, should be obtained.

Collecting Payments

When payments are received for services rendered, the system is working. All collections must be posted to the individual patient's account by the one-step entry manual method or on the computer. Additionally, when posting payments, the account is adjusted for money not received and no longer expected. Adjustments occur when the bill is higher than the payment allowed by the insurance carrier, which happens with Workers' Compensation patients, for whom the state sets its own fee schedule. It also happens when the practice waives the portion of the bill not paid by the insurance company. When providing services to a fellow health professional it is common to provide the colleague with a courtesy discount. By posting collections and writing off the adjustments, the private practice maintains an accurate record of its accounts receivable.

Communicating with Insurance Companies

Frequently problems arise when awaiting payment from insurance companies, which may deny payment or be slow in reimbursement. In either situation someone from the practice must contact the insurance carrier, preferably by telephone in most cases, and should ask to speak with the person in charge of the claim to learn the status of the claim and whether additional information is needed. Any required additional information should be mailed promptly to the person handling the claim. Furthermore, when problems arise with insurance companies, it is a good idea to speak with the claims person's supervisor. The private practice employee who deals with the insurance companies should maintain a file (such as a Rolodex) containing information on each company, including company name, address, telephone number, and, most importantly, key contact person. Although communications with the insurance companies may be frustrating, it will usually prove helpful to handle them in a polite, friendly manner.

Bank Deposits

When payments are actually received from patients and insurance companies and posted to the patients' accounts, the money should be deposited in the practice's checking account. It is most convenient for tracking and accounting purposes to make deposits daily, or at least to fill out a new deposit slip for each day. This will allow for cross-checking the deposits credited by the bank with the amounts listed in the checkbook register. In addition to deposits, payroll taxes must be paid to the bank with the tax coupon for forwarding to the government.

Generating Reports

Report generation is a task for the administrative staff, but is an unrealistic task for noncomputerized private practices. Through the use of computerized software reports can be generated efficiently and accurately. These reports inform the owners of the status of the practice. Some subjects of the reports are: aged accounts, listed by patient; referrals, listed by physician; patient visits, listed by therapist; and patients, listed by insurance company.

SUMMARY

This chapter discusses the many professional and administrative activities that must be competently handled for a private practice to be successful. The number of tasks involved is normally greater than the number of employees in the practice; therefore, in each practice the various tasks will be assigned at the discretion of the owner(s).

SUGGESTED READINGS

Brimer MA: Fundamentals of Private Practice In Physical Therapy. Charles C Thomas, Springfield, IL, 1988
Gazaway JR: Administrative assistant: A valuable asset in your private practice. Whirlpool 10(4):26–27, 1987

Johnston BE, Lord PJ: Your Private Practice. Vol. 2. Planning and Organization. Ben E Johnston Jr & Peter J Lord, Lake City, FL, 1982

O'Mullan P: Reflections of an administrative assistant. Phys Ther Today 11(1):37–38, 1988

US Department of Health and Human Services: International Classification of Diseases. 9th Revision (2nd Ed) Vols. 1–3. Public Health Service-Health Care Financing Administration, Washington, DC, 1980

Young CR: Making Your Practice Grow—A Useful Guide for the Health Care Professional. Bracey Publishing Co., Farmington Hills, MI, 1984

9

THE BUDGET

The budget is one of the most important components of the business management process. Overspending can lead to the lack of necessary cash required to keep the physical therapy practice viable. On the other hand, underspending is often reflected in a poor appearance of the office or a lack of efficiency in collections. A budget is the mechanism for controlling the financial management of the practice.

Part of the responsibility of a private practitioner is financial management. To assist in this function a private practitioner should retain an accountant (see Ch. 4). The cost of an accountant is far less than the cost of incorrect preparation or late filing of tax returns.

A budget is in reality a monthly estimate of revenues and expenditures for the year. By making monthly predictions the manager can assess periodically whether the practice is operating on target. A written report should be generated at least once a month, and adjustments will need to be made to rectify any variance.

Budgets are prepared on a fiscal year basis. This means that a company can choose the 12-month cycle that it wants to use as its yearly accounting cycle, also known as the *tax year*. The fiscal year does not have to correspond to the January to December calendar year, although many private practices do use the calendar year cycle. Accountants can recommend which fiscal year is best.

The budget is a financial portrait of what will be needed to achieve the facility's goals. Once the goals have been established and a plan of action has been formulated, the budget can be prepared. There are basically two types of budgets that are used in the private practice setting: the capital equipment budget and the operating budget. For the new business there is also the preopening budget.

THE PREOPENING BUDGET

The preopening budget is a financial plan that includes any capital equipment outlays and any operating expenses expected to be incurred before opening the

123

facility. The term *capital equipment* usually implies any single piece of equipment that costs over $500 or a quantity of identical items whose aggregate cost exceeds $500. Thus capital equipment includes most physical therapy equipment and major furniture. *Operating expenses* include all salaries, any construction work, hookup fees, promotional expenses (before opening), and any other expenses relating to the operation of the business. Other examples are consulting fees, postage, legal and accounting fees, license fees, minor equipment, office supplies, and training and education costs. It is important to budget so as to give the new business a guideline on spending. A careful tally must be kept to make sure that the funds are still available because enough capital should remain liquid for the first 6 months of operation to ensure that there are enough funds to pay employee salaries and other operating expenses. Capital is considered *liquid* if it is readily accessible for use.

A smart planner will calculate all preopening costs before making the commitment to go into private practice. The requirements for up front money can then be determined. The major reason for business failure is lack of sufficient cash to pay the bills. The preopening costs are often underestimated and need to be addressed thoroughly (see Ch. 3).

CHECKLIST: SAMPLE PREOPENING BUDGET (WITHOUT DOLLAR AMOUNTS)

Construction	_____	Computer and software	_____
Telephone system	_____	Accounting and legal costs	_____
Water meter and sewer hookup	_____	Carpeting/tile	_____
Physical therapy equipment	_____	Advertising/opening announcements	_____
Office and waiting room equipment/ furniture	_____	Marketing	_____
Telephone deposit	_____	_____	_____
Utility deposit	_____	Total	_____

CAPITAL EQUIPMENT BUDGET

Many private practitioners buy a piece of equipment when it is needed. However, if a manager can plan for that need, appropriate funds can be allocated in advance. Facilities with more than one therapist should involve everyone in the decision making process since the equipment will probably be used by all.

The first step in selecting equipment is to determine what type is needed. If another therapist is soon to be employed, the manager may need to order another treatment table. If the practice is merely expanding its office hours, perhaps another table cannot be justified. In the hospital setting, department heads often list the pros and cons of each piece of equipment under consideration; this is a good idea for the private practitioner also.

Second, the private practitioner should determine the approximate number of procedures for which the equipment will be used over the next 5 years. This will help ensure that the purchase of a particular piece of equipment is warranted. For example, a practice may be interested in buying an ultrasound machine. If this machine will be used on 25 percent of the patients and 16 patients are treated per day, then four procedures per day will be generated by the ultrasound machine. If the practice is open 5 days per week, this amounts to 20 procedures per week, or 1,040 per year. Then the estimated charge should be multiplied by the number of procedures to obtain the gross revenue projection for that piece of equipment. If the charge is $20 per procedure, the gross revenue projection would be 1,040 procedures times $20, which equals $20,800 for the first year. During the second year the manager may expect to bring in an additional therapist and use the machine 10 times per day, which amounts to 50 procedures per week and 2,600 for the year. The $20 charge multiplied by 2,600 procedures equals $52,000 for the year. Forecasting should be continued for the next 3 years. Care must be exercised not to overestimate the maximum number of times this machine can be used during a normal workday.

Third, at least three quotes on the exact model or a similar model of the equipment should be obtained. Often manufacturers will grant exclusive dealerships to vendors in certain geographic locations, and therefore only one quote for a particular model may be obtainable. Sometimes the manager needs to select a similar model instead. When computing total cost, it is necessary to include sales tax, shipping charge, vendor installation cost (if any), and cost of any plant modification that may be required. If trading in another piece of equipment, the trade-in value is deducted.

Finally, the financial projections can be made in summary. Number of procedures multiplied by charge per procedure will equal gross revenue for the piece of capital equipment. Subtracting the operating expenses from the gross revenue will give a projection of the gross profit. An example of a capital equipment worksheet is given in Figure 9-1 to facilitate the calculations.

The lifetime of capital equipment varies, and it is important to estimate the longevity and report this to the accountant. Capital equipment can be depreciated over time, that is, part of the equipment cost is transferred from assets to operating expenses and written off each month. For example, if the new capital

CAPITAL EQUIPMENT

Equipment Name _____

Equipment Description _____

_____

_____

_____

Manufacturer _____

Make and Model Number _____

Equipment Pros and Cons

	Pro	Con	Neutral
Price _____			
Warranty _____			
Features _____			
1. _____			
2. _____			
3. _____			
4. _____			
5. _____			
Appearance _____			
Ease of operation _____			
Service contract _____			
Obtainable _____			
Cost _____			
Ease of cleaning _____			
TOTAL:	_____	_____	_____

(continued)

Fig. 9-1. Capital equipment worksheet.

Cost Information

Estimated Equipment Cost

   Price   _____

   Sales tax   _____

   Shipping cost   _____

   Installation fee   _____

   Inservice fee   _____

                  Estimated cost   _____

                  Less trade-in   _____

TOTAL ESTIMATED EQUIPMENT COST   _____

Estimated Plant Modifications

   Electrical   _____

   Heating/AC   _____

   Plumbing   _____

   Other   _____

TOTAL ESTIMATED PLANT MODIFICATIONS   _____

PLUS TOTAL ESTIMATED EQUIPMENT COST   _____

TOTAL ESTIMATED COST   _____

Financial Projections

REVENUE	Year 1	2	3	4	5
No. of procedures	___	___	___	___	___
Charge per procedure	___	___	___	___	___
Gross revenue	___	___	___	___	___
DIRECT OPERATING EXPENSES					
Salaries, wages, & benefits	___	___	___	___	___
Repairs & maintenance	___	___	___	___	___
Supplies & linen	___	___	___	___	___
Other	___	___	___	___	___
Total Expenses	___	___	___	___	___
GROSS PROFIT	___	___	___	___	___

Fig. 9-1. (*continued*)

equipment in the physical therapy practice cost $120,000 and can be depreciated over a 10-year period, then $12,000 per year, or $1,000 per month, can be charged to the depreciation account.

OPERATING BUDGET

The next type of budget that needs to be addressed is the operating budget, which contains the categories of expenses not included in the capital equipment budget. In a physical therapy private practice, the operating budget should be a *flexible budget* (i.e., one that is based on cost per unit of service and is therefore volume-dependent). Although this type of budget will not always be accurate because of shortages of professional staff in many areas, it can serve the private practitioner well if temporary personnel can be used until a clear need for an additional therapist exists. Operating budgets have both a revenue and an expense side.

Revenues

In the physical therapy practice, *revenue* is the total dollar amount billed for the visits. Revenue is projected based on visits or units of service per month. A *visit* is considered one total outpatient treatment for a particular day. A *unit of service*, on the other hand, is normally thought of as a procedure, such as ultrasound, exercise, or cold pack. One can project revenues based either on average charge per visit (e.g., $60) or on charge per unit of service (e.g., $20 for each procedure). It is good to keep track of both, but for the purposes of this book the sample budget will be based on visits.

It is difficult to project visits before opening, but most facilities start with one therapist and work from there. An orthopedically oriented private practice may proceed on the assumption that a therapist can handle 15 visits per day. In a facility that is neurologically oriented it may be felt that 8 to 10 visits are all that one therapist can manage. Future trends may be based on past volumes (e.g., if the practice has had a 25 percent increase in volume for each of the last 3 years, the same may be expected for the next fiscal year). Usually growth is not this easily predictable. More often it is related to various factors which include: reputation; other private practices in the area; current trends among physicians, such as health maintenance organizations, preferred provider organizations and physician-owned physical therapy services; degree of specialization; personality of the therapists; and marketing efforts. If a new program such as work hardening is marketed successfully, an increase in visit projections is warranted. One can also ask area physicians, rehabilitation specialists, etc. for an estimate of how many of certain types of patients they see to decide whether they are likely to refer all or some of their patients to the physical therapy practice.

Charges can be established by several methods. One method is to find out what the other area private practices are charging, but the best way is to determine the costs per patient visit or procedure and then estimate what profit the practice requires.

Cost per Visit

To obtain an overall picture of the true costs of a visit, the time required for each visit including preparations, setup, actual treatment, and cleanup and charting time must be calculated (see Fig. 9-2). Then salary, wages, and benefits (SW&B) per minute for each visit and any expenses for supplies (e.g., ultrasound gel and linen) are calculated. An overhead allocation to cover all the indirect costs relating to a visit is added (e.g., administrative and clerical costs, including salaries and supplies). Depreciation per procedure can be calculated by dividing the cost of the equipment by the number of years over which it is being depreciated (usually 5 to 10 years, depending on the piece of equipment) and then dividing it by the number of procedures expected over its useful life. An accountant can be consulted to assist in determining the appropriate number of years to be depreciated based on the useful life of the equipment.

Expenses

Expenses are any costs a facility incurs in rendering its services; they can be classified as fixed or variable. *Fixed expenses* remain constant for a given time frame (e.g., rent and salaries). Salaries are used here to indicate financial remuneration paid to those personnel making a fixed salary that does not fluctuate with hours or volume of work. *Variable expenses,* those that vary in direct proportion to the volume produced, include medical and office supplies and the wages of hourly staff and per diem staff (those personnel who work only the number of hours the facility needs). Their hourly rates are usually higher than those of regular employees, but they are not normally paid any benefits. Per diem staff help to keep the wage expense account down during volume fluctuations, which occur in many parts of the United States depending on the time of the year. For example, many parts of Florida experience seasonal fluctuations, the summer being slow and the winter extraordinarily busy.

As previously stated, it is important to know costs per visit. Even fixed costs can be spread over a period of time based on the visit or volume projections. For example, if the practice's volume is 1,000 visits per month and the rent is $3,000, the expense for rent is $3 per visit per month. Variable expenses can vary monthly, but when the total yearly volume is divided into the total yearly costs, an average cost per visit can be calculated for the year. For example, in May the total variable expenses may be $15,000 for 600 visits, which means that the variable expenses are $25 per visit. For the year, however, the total variable expenses may be $180,000 for 6,000 visits, or $30 per visit. Even though the costs change, they are still the same for all procedures within a given time frame. Figure 9–3 graphically depicts fixed and variable expenses.

COST PER VISIT

	SW&B per minute	x	Total minutes	=	Total SW&B	+	Other Expenses	=	Total

Preparation

Reading chart   ____   ____   ____   ____   ____

Speaking with

physician   ____   ____   ____   ____   ____

Other   ____   ____   ____   ____   ____

Setup

Greeting patient, leading to treatment area, giving gown, helping onto plinth

                       ____   ____   ____   ____   ____

Linen costs

  Towels   ____   ____   ____   ____   ____

  Washclothes ____   ____   ____   ____   ____

  Sheets   ____   ____   ____   ____   ____

Supply costs

  1.   ____   ____

  2.   ____   ____

  3.   ____   ____

Actual Treatment

Equipment depreciation   ____   ____

Actual treatment time   ____   ____   ____   ____   ____

Cleanup and Charting

Cleanup   ____   ____   ____   ____   ____

Charting   ____   ____   ____   ____   ____

Correspondence   ____   ____   ____   ____   ____

Other Overhead (Taken as a % of Total Costs)

                       ____   ____   ____   ____   ____

Cost per Visit   ____   ____   ____   ____   ____

TOTAL COSTS FOR ABOVE VISIT   _____

Fig. 9-2. Cost per procedure worksheet.

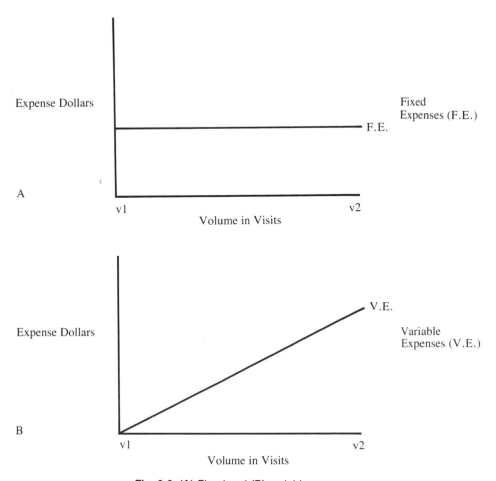

Fig. 9-3. (A) Fixed and **(B)** variable expenses.

Chart of Accounts

Initially it is quite difficult to estimate costs. The best method is to formulate a *chart of accounts,* which is a listing of those revenue and expense categories that are pertinent to the business. The physical therapy private practitioner may want either to have one chart of accounts for the entire facility or to break it down by area (e.g., administration and physical therapy clinical services). The latter is an excellent way to determine *overhead* costs (any that are not directly related to patient care) versus direct clinical expense. Overhead expenses include rent, office supplies, postage, etc.

For multidisciplinary private practices, the chart of accounts for the revenue side would have physical therapy revenue, speech/language pathology revenue, etc. In many private practice settings there will be only one revenue account,

Table 9-1. Chart of Accounts

Administration	Clinical Services
Regular hours	Regular hours
Overtime hours	Overtime hours
Vacation/holiday	Vacation/holiday
Sick pay	Sick pay
Payroll taxes and insurance	Payroll taxes and insurance
Group insurance	Group insurance
Pension, retirement	Pension, retirement
Rent	Medical supplies
Office supplies and expense	Office supplies and expense
Repairs and maintenance	Repairs and maintenance
Service contracts	Service contracts
Postage and freight	Equipment rental
License and fees	Travel and education
Equipment rental	Minor equipment
Travel and education	Dues and subscriptions
Dues and subscriptions	Linen
Utilities	
Electrical	
Water	
Telephone	
Other	
Advertising	
Consulting fees	
Housekeeping supplies	
Loan payment	

patient revenue (unless the practitioner chooses to have separate revenue accounts for each specialty program).

Table 9-1 shows expenses for both administration and clinical services as they would be listed in a chart of accounts.

Sample Operating Budget

Once the chart of accounts is established, the manager can proceed with preparation of the operating budget. Typically, the number of visits per month for the fiscal year is predicted, and the average charge per visit is then multiplied by the anticipated number of visits to obtain the gross revenue (see Table 9-2).

Staffing

Staffing is estimated by using *full-time equivalents (FTE)*. One FTE equals 40 hours of work per week. *Nonproductive hours* are any hours during the week for which the employee is paid but does not actually work, such as sick time and vacation hours. *Productive hours* are those hours during which the employee actually works, including regular and overtime hours. An example is shown in Table 9-3 for a facility that opened with two therapists and one secretary (i.e., 2.0 physical therapist FTEs and 1.0 secretary FTE).

Table 9-2. Estimating Revenue Fiscal Year 19——

	Jan.	Feb.	Mar.	Apr.	May	June	July	Aug.	Sep.	Oct.	Nov.	Dec.	Total for Year
No. of visits	488	650	812	650	650	650	650	650	600	550	700	750	7800
Average charge ($)/ visit	60	60	60	60	60	60	60	60	60	60	60	60	60
Gross revenue ($)/ month	29,280	39,000	48,720	39,000	39,000	39,000	39,000	39,000	36,000	33,000	42,000	45,000	468,000

Table 9-3. Estimating Staffing Requirements (FTEs)

	Jan.	Feb.	Mar.	Apr.	May	June	July	Aug.	Sep.	Oct.	Nov.	Dec.	Total
Physical therapists	2.0	2.5	2.5	2.5	2.5	2.5	2.5	2.5	2.5	2.5	2.8	3.0	2.53
Secretary	1.0	1.0	1.0	1.5	1.5	1.5	1.5	1.5	1.5	1.5	1.5	1.5	1.38

The above staffing pattern is only semiflexible, but as the facility grows, staffing can become more flexible. Flexibility also depends on the availability of contract, part-time, or per diem labor. There are 2,080 hours in a year as far as employee productive and nonproductive hours are concerned; therefore, the average number of employee hours in a month is 173.33 per FTE (2,080 hours divided by 12 months equals 173.33). Thus, depending on the average amount of time spent per patient per visit, a flexible staffing pattern can be calculated for the facility.

Wages, Salaries, and Benefits

For the FTEs considered above, Table 9-4 provides an example of the productive and nonproductive hours that could be budgeted for the physical therapists, as well as the wage, salary, and benefit expenses. The manager will want to keep overtime hours to a minimum, but they are given here to illustrate a possibility that might arise in a given month. The total hours are calculated by multiplying the number of employees by 173.33 hours per month (based on an 8-hour day), and projected vacation, sick, holiday hours, etc. that can be expected are then subtracted to obtain total productive hours. Regular hours are productive hours that do not exceed 40 per week. Overtime is paid to any employee who works over 40 hours per week and is not salaried, since salaried workers are considered to be exempt from receiving overtime and are usually professional people. Whether to pay the employees wages (hourly employees) plus overtime when appropriate or to pay them a salary (i.e., a set amount per period of time, such as $35,000 per year) but no overtime is a personal decision. Employees who are salaried at the above rate and paid weekly would be paid a gross salary (salary before taxes) of $673.08 per week ($35,000 divided by 52) no matter how many hours they worked in the week. The average hourly rate used here is purely arbitrary—the rate is normally based on experience and regional variations.

Payroll taxes and insurance includes FICA (Social Security tax), federal unemployment tax, state unemployment tax, and Workers' Compensation insurance. Health insurance rates can vary tremendously depending on the age and number of the employees, the regional location, and sometimes whether or not the employees are smokers (see Table 9-4).

All the nonsalary operating budget costs are based on a set cost per visit, which will vary from facility to facility depending on how the owners wish to spend their money. For the above clinic, medical expenses were based on approximately 29 cents per visit (see Table 9-2 for projected visits), and office supplies were based on about 35 cents per visit. A sample nonsalary operating budget is depicted in Table 9-5.

Variance Reports

Most private practices tally their total revenues for the month and then deduct total expenses to figure their pretax income. The variance report lists each item in the chart of accounts. Each account listed is referred to as a *line item*; for

Table 9-4. Wages, Salaries, and Benefits

	Jan.	Feb.	Mar.	Apr.	May	June	July	Aug.	Sep.	Oct.	Nov.	Dec.	Total
Salary and wages													
Regular hours	331	433	433	418	398	418	377	394	381	393	417	460	4,853
Overtime hours	0	0	0	5	0	0	4	0	0	0	4	4	17
Total productive hours	331	433	433	423	398	418	381	394	381	393	421	464	4,870
Total productive FTEs	1.9	2.5	2.5	2.4	2.3	2.4	2.2	2.3	2.2	2.3	2.4	2.7	2.3
Vacation hours	0	0	0	0	0	0	8	16	16	16	16	24	96
Holiday hours	16	0	0	0	20	0	20	0	20	8	16	24	124
Sick pay hours	0	0	0	8	8	2	8	8	8	8	16	0	66
Education hours	0	0	0	2	8	8	16	16	8	8	16	8	90
Total nonproductive hours	16	0	0	10	36	10	52	40	52	40	64	56	376
Total nonproductive FTEs	0.1	0	0	0.1	0.2	0.1	0.3	0.2	0.3	0.2	0.4	0.3	0.2
Total FTEs	2.0	2.5	2.5	2.5	2.5	2.5	2.5	2.5	2.5	2.5	2.8	3.0	2.53
Total hours	347	433	433	433	434	433	433	434	433	433	485	520	5,246
Avg. hourly rate	15.65	15.65	15.65	15.65	15.65	15.65	15.65	15.65	15.65	15.65	15.65	15.65	15.65
Avg. overtime rate	23.48	23.48	23.48	23.48	23.48	23.48	23.48	23.48	23.48	23.48	23.48	23.48	23.48
Total salaries and wages	5,431	6,776	6,776	6,817	6,792	6,776	6,808	6,792	6,776	6,776	7,622	8,232	82,233
Payroll taxes and insurance ($)	434	542	542	546	543	542	545	544	542	542	610	659	6,579
Health insurance ($)	272	339	339	341	340	339	340	340	339	339	381	412	4,112
Total salaries, wages, and benefits ($)	6,137	7,657	7,657	7,704	7,675	7,657	7,693	7,676	7,657	7,657	8,613	9,303	92,924

Table 9-5. Nonsalary Operating Budget

	Jan.	Feb.	Mar.	Apr.	May	June	July	Aug.	Sep.	Oct.	Nov.	Dec.	Total
Medical supplies	122	163	203	163	163	163	163	163	150	138	175	188	2,239
Office supplies	171	228	284	228	228	228	228	228	210	193	245	263	2,734
Minor equipment	50	50	100	50	50	50	50	50	100	50	50	50	700
Service contracts	42	42	42	42	42	42	42	42	42	42	42	42	504
Travel and education	500	500	500	500	500	500	500	500	500	500	500	500	6,000
Dues and subscriptions	50	50	50	50	0	0	0	0	0	0	0	750	950
Repairs and maintenance	160	160	160	160	160	160	160	160	160	160	160	160	160
Total nonsalary operating costs	1,095	1,143	1,339	1,193	1,143	1,143	1,143	1,143	1,162	1,083	1,172	1,953	13,287

Table 9-6. Variance Report, Month Ending ...., 19xx

Description	Actual	Budget	Percent Variance
Revenue			
No. of patient visits	1,500	1,800	(16.6)
Revenue per visit	60	60	0
Patient revenue	90,000	108,000	(16.6)
Expenses			
Salary and wages			
Regular hours	800	960	(16.6)
Regular dollars	12,000	15,000	(16.6)
Overtime hours	10	5	100
Overtime dollars	120	60	100
Subtotal Productive hours/ dollars	810	965	(16.0)
Subtotal Productive Dollars	12,620	15,060	(16.2)
Productive Hours per Visit	.54	.54	0
Productive dollars per visit	8.33	8.37	0.4
Productive FTEs	5.1	6.0	(15.0)
Vacation hours	20.0	40.0	50
Vacation dollars	313.00	625.00	50
Holiday hours	40.0	40.0	0
Holiday dollars	625.00	625.00	0
Sick pay hours	0	8	(100)
Sick pay dollars	0	125.00	(100)
Subtotal Nonproductive hours	60	88	(31.8)
Subtotal Nonproductive dollars	938.00	1,375.00	(31.8)
Total salary and wage hours	870	1,053	(17.3)
Total salary and wage dollars	13,558	16,435	(17.3)
Total hours/visit	0.58	0.58	0
Total FTEs	5.44	6.55	(16.9)
Payroll taxes and insurance	1,085	1,315	(17.5)
Health insurance	678	822	(17.5)
Medical supplies	375	450	(16.6)
Office supplies	525	630	(16.6)
Minor equipment	150	100	50
Service contracts	75	100	(25)
Travel and education	800	1,000	(20)
Dues and subscriptions	200	200	0
Repairs and maintenance	40	50	(20)
Total direct expense	17,486	21,102	(17)
Total direct expenses per visit	11.66	11.72	(.5)
Income before indirect expenses	72,514	86,898	(16.6)
Margin on gross revenue	80.6%	80.5%	0.1

example, medical supplies is a line item and so is rent. Each actual line item is compared with the budgeted amounts and the percent variance is calculated. A condensed sample variance report is shown in Table 9-6.

Productive hours per visit equal the amount of time spent by the staff (professional and nonprofessional) per patient visit, while nonproductive hours are vacation, holiday, education, and sick hours that are spent out of the office but must be paid out as benefits and are therefore charged per patient visit. Productive and nonproductive hours per visit add up to total hours per visit. The figures given are based on an 8-hour day. For example, if a therapist is paid for 8 hours a day and treats 15 patients in that time, the average total time spent with each patient is 0.53 hour.

Total direct expenses per visit are those amounts spent directly on patient care, whereas indirect expenses are considered overhead (see Figure 9-2). The *gross margin* is the excess of revenue over direct expenses in each department. In the case above, the gross margin is profit before deducting all other indirect expenses, such as rent and administrative costs.

OTHER ACCOUNTING PRINCIPLES

Economic resources owned by the business are called *assets*, and the owner's investments are called *owner's equity*. The debts of the company are referred to as *liabilities*. The following accounting equation shows the relationship among these three concepts.

Assets = liabilities + owner's equity

Any business transaction that takes place in the private practice affects these three elements.

Assets can include cash, land, equipment, accounts receivable, notes receivable, and prepaid expenses. *Current assets* are any assets that will be converted to cash or used up within a year. *Fixed assets* are those that are relatively permanent and can be depreciated over time, such as building and equipment. *Accounts receivable* is a term used to designate revenue owed by patients or third party payers. *Notes receivable* are more formal and require a written statement of the amount and date the note is to be paid. Any time that the word *receivable* is used, an asset is being discussed. *Prepaid expenses* include inventory and any payments made in advance, such as professional liability insurance.

Liabilities are those debts that the business owes to other people or businesses. If ultrasound gel is purchased on credit, it is posted to *accounts payable.* Whenever the term *payable* is used, it implies a liability. *Current liabilities,* like current assets, fall due in a year or less. These include notes payable, accounts payable, taxes payable, and salaries and wages payable. On the other hand, *long-term* liabilities are those due after more than 1 year (e.g., a mortgage to be paid in a lump sum at the end of 5 years would be a long-term liability classified as a mortgage note payable).

Owner's equity is often referred to as shareholder's or stockholder's equity. For the sole proprietor, partnership, or professional association, owner's equity is sometimes called *net worth.* When the business is a corporation, the investment of the shareholders is called *capital stock,* and *retained earnings* are that portion of the net income kept in the business.

Business transactions are initially entered into a book called a *journal*, which provides a permanent record of increases and decreases in an account. The journalized entries are then periodically transferred to the ledger, in which a complete record of all the company's accounts are kept and the *trial balance* is verified. The trial balance is a calculation to check that debits equal credits. Debits and credits are increases or decreases in an account (see discussion of the chart of accounts).

There are three major accounting statements that are used to communicate the financial positions of the private practice. The first is the *income statement,* also known as the profit and loss (P & L) statement (Figure 9-4). This statement summarizes the revenues and expenses for a defined period of time, sometimes monthly but at least quarterly and annually. The second statement is the *statement of owner's equity*, which provides a summary of any changes in owner's equity, such as could result from expenses, revenues, owner's investments, or withdrawals. Like the income statement, the statement of owner's equity is prepared for defined periods of time, but at least annually. The third statement, the *balance sheet* (Fig. 9-5) depicts the assets, liabilities, and owner's equity of the practice as of a stated date, usually the end of the fiscal year. Normally an accountant would provide these statements for the business after a review of the records.

BUDGET CHECKLIST

Preopening budget	____	Operating budget and chart of accounts	____
Capital equipment budget—type of equipment, number of procedures per machine, quotes on equipment	____	Variance reports	____
Fixed and variable expenses	____	Assets, liabilities, and stockholder's equity	____
		Income statement	____
		Balance sheet	____

SUMMARY

This chapter has focused on the financial aspects of physical therapy private practice. A knowledge of basic accounting principles is important for the smooth functioning of the facility. Budgeting is a management function that allows

Company X
Income Statement
For Year Ended June 30, 19xx

REVENUES		$450,000
Operating Expenses		
Salaries, wages, & benefits	$155,000	
Rent	43,200	
Medical supplies	1,600	
Non-medical supplies	1,200	
Telephone & utilities	7,550	
Insurance	3,500	
Office expenses	4,800	
Advertising	6,500	
Accounting & legal	5,500	
Depreciation	13,500	
Amortization	2,100	
Licenses & taxes	400	
Travel & education	6,000	
Dues & subscriptions	750	
Loan interest & principal payments	25,000	
Maintenance	600	
Miscellaneous	2,000	
TOTAL OPERATING EXPENSES		$279,200
Pretax Income		170,800
Income Taxes		43,200
NET INCOME		127,600

Fig. 9-4. Sample income statement.

Company X
Balance Sheet
December 31, 19xx

ASSETS

Current assets

Cash	$23,000	
Accounts receivable	38,000	
Inventory	800	
Prepaid expense	3,000	
		$64,800

Fixed assets

Equipment	$135,000	
Accumulated depreciation	(35,000)	100,000
		$164,800

LIABILITIES AND OWNER'S EQUITY

Current liabilities

Accounts Payable	$5,600	
Income Taxes Payable	3,220	$8,820

Owner's Equity

J. Jones, capital	$155,980
	$164,800

Fig. 9-5. Sample balance sheet.

forecasting by standardized techniques and refocusing as needed after an analysis of the monthly variance report. Although an accountant should prepare the financial statements, time and money are saved by setting up the appropriate financial systems at the start. Knowing how to read the financial statements will also allow the practitioner to ask educated questions and spare the accountant from being asked a multitude of irrelevant ones.

SUGGESTED READINGS

Bacon J: Managing the Budget Function. The Conference Board, Inc., New York, 1973

Byars LL: Concepts of Strategic Management, Planning and Implementation. Harper & Row, New York, 1984

Fess E, Warren CS: Accounting Principles. South-Western Publishing Co., Cincinnati, 1987

Horngren CT: Cost Accounting, A Managerial Emphasis. Prentice-Hall, Englewood Cliffs, NJ, 1982

10

MARKETING

Marketing the physical therapy private practice can be one of the most interesting aspects of the management of the business. Strategic planning and the implementation of the marketing plans play an important role in the success of the practice. The entire staff—secretary, manager, physical therapists, and all other employees—are responsible for a certain amount of marketing every day. If the private practice is not able to have a marketing manager, then the facility administrator or senior physical therapist must manage the marketing activities to ensure that the organization achieves its goals and objectives.

Most marketing experts cite product, place, promotion, and price, the four Ps, as the major components of marketing.

PRODUCT

The *product* in the physical therapy private practice is the performance of the physical therapy service itself. (If goods such as lumbar rolls, weights, and hot or cold packs are sold they are also included in this category.) "Packaging" the physical therapy product is important. The inside and outside appearance of the facility can either attract or deter clients. The facility should always be clean and neat and look professional. Equipment should be cleaned frequently and kept in good repair. Likewise, staff should appear well-groomed and be friendly and professional in their manner.

The channel of distribution, moving the product to the final customer, is quite complex in the manufacturing industry. However, it is very simple for the physical therapy private practice; the product moves directly from the producer to the customer, that is, from the therapist to the patient.

PLACE

The design and location of the *place* has been discussed in Chapters 5 and 6. The marketability of the place involves providing service in an area where it is wanted and needed. For example, opening a practice near a facility where all the physicians have their own physical therapists on staff can lead to the new practice's quick demise.

PROMOTION

Promotion involves informing the target market, those homogeneous groups of customers to whom the company wishes to appeal, about the physical therapy services available. For the physical therapy private practice, the target market may include back and neck, pediatric, or cardiac rehabilitation clients. Submarkets include anyone who can refer a client: physicians, social workers, rehabilitation specialists, industries, as well as insurance carriers. Promotion uses the concepts of personal selling, mass selling, and sales promotion.

Personal Selling

Personal selling is direct one-on-one contact between the marketer and someone in the target market or sub-markets. Personal selling occurs between every patient and therapist as treatment is rendered, and between patient and other staff members because a patient has the ability to refer friends, relatives, and neighbors to the practice. Personal selling usually involves meeting with physicians who can refer patients to the business and explaining to them the services offered and the expertise of the staff. Meeting with social workers in the community, insurance adjusters, personnel directors, employee health physicians and nurses, and other allied health professionals will stimulate referrals. Maintaining contact via correspondence, phone calls, and intermittent personal visits can build the rapport needed to develop referral patterns.

Mass Selling

Mass selling usually involves reaching out to large numbers of customers, either through advertising or publicity. *Advertising* refers to any paid form of business representation, such as radio, billboards, television, magazines, or flyers. *Publicity*, on the other hand, is a nonpaid form of business representation (e.g., a therapist appearing as a guest speaker on television or a newspaper story about one of the practice's patients who has done well).

Advertising can be very expensive, so the administrator must determine which media are best suited to the practice's needs. Every private practice should advertise at least in the telephone yellow pages. Also, the business should have its name, address, and phone number listed in as many other directories as possible, especially in its primary and secondary service areas. Many organizations—the local medical society, chamber of commerce, mayor's committee for the disabled, and county service directories—will list the practice for free. Furthermore, if the therapists in the practice join the American Physical Therapy Association (APTA), they can be listed in the local and state directories. If staff members join an APTA section, such as the Private Practice Section, they will be listed in its directory.

Announcements in the local newspapers are an excellent way of informing the public of such events as the opening of the practice, additions of staff, and expansion of services and hours. These announcements should be made periodically to obtain name exposure. Radio advertising is a good possibility, depending on the market area. Billboards and bench advertising are being used more frequently, but billboard advertising in prime locations can be expensive. One of the more effective means of advertising is having a sign outside the facility that can be seen from the street. The sign should be eye catching yet professional in appearance. Magazine and television advertising are not generally used by the small business.

Direct mailings are very effective and should be done at least once a month. They can be in the form of a letter on the business's stationery, a newsletter, referral pads, business cards, Rolodex telephone directory cards, Christmas cards, announcements, company or program brochures, and newspaper reprints about the company or one of the patients. Such direct mailings are sent to physicians, attorneys, industry, rehabilitation specialists, insurance carriers, community agencies, support groups, physician office managers, among others. Mailing lists can be purchased through local marketing companies, or the practice can come up with its own lists. The yellow pages is a good place to start.

Sales Promotion

Sales promotion consists of revenue-generating activities that are not considered personal or mass selling. It includes trade shows, conventions, professional association meetings, guest lectures, business or civic group meetings, open houses, and health fairs and group discount plans for local businesses. Group discount plans are commonly available in the industrial medicine and executive physical departments of many hospitals. Executive physical departments offer comprehensive physical examinations (including cardiac stress tests) to corporate executives.

Public Relations

Public relations is another form of promotion. City or town officials should be invited to the practice to become acquainted with its services. Local government officials can often suggest more contacts that might be interested in the facility's services. A contract could be worked out with the city to give a discount to its employees requiring physical therapy services (see sales promotion above). State and federal legislators should also hear the practice's voice on political issues.

Public relations also includes getting involved with the community: joining the local Chamber of Commerce, Rotary Club, Lion's Club, and other civic organizations. The local mayor's committee for the disabled, the YMCA, the regional office of the Paralyzed Veterans of America, other organizations with "special olympic" events, the local Arthritis Foundation, or the American Heart Association can all be served through physical therapy services or by volunteering to assist the organization's particular need. There are many more special interest groups—organizations dedicated to a special cause—that need help (e.g., the American Physical Therapy Association, dedicated to the enhancement of the physical therapy profession; the Chamber of Commerce, concerned with commerce on a local, state, and national level). These interest groups, and many more, can usually be found in the yellow pages under "associations." In general, the more people who know the staff and the name of the business, the better the chance of patient referrals.

Patient Relations

Patient relations, another form of sales promotion, includes all communication between the practice's staff members and patients. A warm, friendly atmosphere will make people want to come back. Any employee who does not smile and speak courteously to the patients and their families or visitors should not be employed. Even the person who collects money must always be professional and helpful. The receptionist should greet each patient and visitor. An offer of a cup of coffee or soda helps break down any uneasiness the patient may feel. All employees who come into contact with a patient should introduce themselves. Correspondence with patients should be carefully worded. Communication involving discrepancies should promote a win-win attitude so that the patient does not become defensive.

One of the most important aspects of good patient relations is to have qualified competent physical therapists. Employing specialists in the practice and having state-of-the-art equipment will develop credibility. Having evening and Saturday hours also promotes good patient relations. Clean lavatory and treatment areas are a must.

Other Types of Promotion

To stimulate referrals, some facilities use giveaways (e.g., coffee mugs, pens, candy, message pads, and paper clip holders). Others send flowers, fruit, balloons, candy, wine, or popcorn to promote referrals or as a gesture of gratitude for existing referrals. Lunches or dinner with individuals is a good way to talk about the business, and group breakfasts, brunches, or lunches at the practice is an excellent way to meet and show the practice to office managers, social workers, and rehabilitation nurses, among other professionals. Having association or community meetings at the office is another excellent marketing strategy. Specific promotional materials will be discussed in the latter part of this chapter.

PRICE

The last of the four Ps, *price,* is especially important in a competitive market. Price is best determined by calculating the facility's expenses, then adding a certain percentage for profit. If the practice is more expensive than the competing practices, the practice may be fostering a no-growth pattern. If the established price does not provide a fair return to the business investors, it is best not to be in business. Therefore, the bottom line should be providing physical therapy services at a competitive rate that gives a fair return on investment.

STRATEGIC PLANNING

At least yearly, every private practice should formulate a written marketing plan that outlines the company's strategy to achieve its marketing goals with specific timeframes. This detailed strategic plan allows the administrator to make operational decisions within certain guidelines and restrictions. For example, a company allots $10,000 to advertising that is expected to cause a 15 percent increase in gross revenue by March 1. If, after spending $5,000, the administrator sees no increase in revenue, then a switch to a different and possibly more effective advertising medium may be needed.

For a sample marketing plan, see Appendices 10-1 and 10-2.

PROMOTIONAL MATERIAL

Everything and every person representing the practice—staff, copy, graphics, media, printing, and decor and appearance—can demonstrate its quality.

Stationery

The practice's image is most frequently presented by its printed materials: letterhead, envelopes, business cards, announcements, referral pads, and patient education pamphlets. All printed items must be consistent with the image the practice wishes to convey. Each item must include the name, location, and phone number of the practice. A corporate logo will provide consistency from one item to the next.

Corporate Logo

A graphic designer should be hired to create a logo based on the corporate name and keywords that best describe the practice. Two or three logos should be created from which to select. When making the final selection, the practice's owners should consider the practice's image, production costs and adaptability from one print medium to another (i.e., not only paper, but also T-shirts, coffee mugs, lumbar rolls, etc.). The owners should remember that production costs are higher when reproducing multiple-colored logos.

Design and Layout

It is preferable that the graphic designer be responsible for designing the layout for stationery as well as the logo. If this is not possible, the graphic designer should provide a camera ready copy of the logo, in a variety of sizes, and the specific Pantone Matching System (PMS) colors to present to the printers.

To design and lay out stationery items, the designer must be provided with the desired copy for each item. Copy for the letterhead includes logo, name of practice, address, phone number, and names of all the partners. Adding therapists who are employees is optional. Copy for a second page of letterhead should be included. Copy for the envelope includes the logo, name of practice, and address. One might consider creating an additional envelope layout with the bulk permit number, if applicable. Copy for the business cards should include the logo, name of practice, address, and a highly visible phone number.

The graphic designer will create separate camera-ready copy for each stationery item. The copy should be thoroughly proofed for typographical errors. The design should be considered for adaptability to both a typewriter and a computer printer.

The final design step is to select the paper stock. The graphic artist should educate the practitioner regarding the advantages and disadvantages of different qualities and colors. The paper stock should be consistent for all major printed materials. The goal is to familiarize the consumer with the practice via regular mailings and correspondence. If the practice's printed materials are inconsistent for each mailing, the consumer is less likely to become familiar with the practice's logo.

CHECKLIST FOR PROMOTIONAL MATERIALS

Essentials		Optional	
Letterhead	____	Informals	____
Second page	____	Announcements	____
Envelopes	____	Invitations	____
Business cards	____	Referral pads	____
Appointment cards	____		

SPECIAL CONSIDERATIONS FOR PROMOTIONAL ITEMS
Business Cards

Distinctively designed business cards can be very advantageous to the practice. They should be visible to everyone who enters the office and should be exchanged during any business conversation with new contacts. Any correspondence with a physician or other contact should include several business cards.

The practice's owners must decide whether to have one business card with all of the partners names included, one business card with all of the partners and therapists' names included, or individual business cards for each professional staff member. (Including all the names associated with a practice allows the consumer to view all of the owners' and/or staff members' credentials together.) Optional information could include office hours, "by appointment only," "referral by physician," and any other personal preferences.

Revolving Card Directories

Since most business offices maintain Rolodex or other type of card directory, the practice could produce a printed card, in plastic or thick paper, for distribution to contacts. The card would resemble the practice's business card. It is a good idea to put physical therapy on the card tab since this is the category under which it should be filed for easy access.

Referral Pads

Referral pads are not only a necessity for prescriptions from doctors, but an effective marketing maneuver. On every marketing call to a physician's office, two pads should be delivered, one for the physician and one for the office manager. This maneuver opens the path of communication between the physician's office and the physical therapy practice. The referral pad also serves as a constant reminder to the physician.

Referral pads should be customized to the practice and encompass state regulations. The practice's owners might decide to have more than one version. For example, a small pad is easier to carry into a referring physician's office, is easier for the physician to fill out, and resembles the medical model of a prescription pad. A larger pad could be used when more space is needed for information (e.g., to fulfill Medicare and Workers' Compensation requirements for referrals).

Brochure

A brochure, a valuable marketing tool, describes the practice in print. It provides ample space to use creative graphics, professional photography, and written copy to educate and establish credibility with the consumer. People need a tangible reminder of the practice, and the brochure serves this purpose. A brochure can bond a new patient to the practice.

Almost every business requires some form of sales literature to keep its products and services in the customer's mind, distinguish itself from the competition, and answer a prospective client's questions. Brochures should be handed out following presentations, given to physicians during marketing calls, distributed during open houses and professional conferences, and mailed to perspective referral sources.

Because of the extensive mileage that a brochure provides, time and money should be spent on its development. A professionally produced brochure should

1. Reflect the image that the practice wants the consumer to feel

2. Provide the reader with the information the practice wants the consumer to know
3. Have a cover that catches the eye and includes the corporate logo
4. Include professional photography that illustrates the key elements of the practice
5. Establish the credibility of the practice

During the brochure's production the practice's representative will be required to contribute information regarding its key elements: paper, color, photographs, size, copy, design and budget. All these elements combined produce the image one wishes to create.

OPEN HOUSE

An open house can be held when the practice first opens, when celebrating an event, or without a particular reason. It is another effective marketing tool for enticing potential clients and referral sources into the office. The incentives are food, entertainment, and possible exposure for the guest. The guest list can include patients past and present, family, friends, equipment vendors, local politicians, colleagues and referral sources (past, current, and potential).

Many offices delay their open house until the practice has been operating for a while, has a more stable clientele and is better equipped. Other practitioners feel the sooner they have the open house the quicker the practice grows. Budgetary constraints must be considered when setting the date. If there is minimal money in the budget for promotion when the office first opens, it may prove beneficial to wait until funds are available for a tastefully done open house rather than a hastily arranged one with inadequate refreshments and poor guest attendance. This would not project a positive image.

SUMMARY

This chapter discusses the development and implementation of a marketing plan for the private physical therapy practice, including some of the promotional materials available and public relations strategies and use of advertising.

SUGGESTED READING

APTA PR Manual For Physical Therapists. American Physical Therapy Association, Alexandria, VA, 1986

Bernstein AL: The Health Professional's Marketing Handbook. Year Book Medical Publishers, Chicago, 1988

Byars, LL: Concepts of Strategic Management, Planning and Implementation. Harper & Row, New York, 1984

Dalrymple DJ, Parsons LJ: Marketing Management Strategy And Cases. John Wiley & Sons, New York, 1986

Davidson, JP: Marketing on a Shoestring, John Wiley & Sons, New York, 1988

Heffernan S: Market research as a tool for the private physical therapy practice. Whirlpool 10(2):34–37, Summer 1987

Jeffries JR, Bates JD: The Executive's Guide To Meetings, Conferences, & Audiovisual Presentations. McGraw-Hill, New York, 1983

McCarthy EJ, Perrault WD Jr: Basic Marketing. Richard D Irwin, Inc., Homewood, IL, 1987

Phillips M & Rasberry S: Marketing Without Advertising. Nolo Press, Berkeley, California, 1986

Poppe F: 50 Rules to Keep a Client Happy. Harper & Row, New York, 1987

Rosenbloom B: Marketing Channels—A Management View. Dryden Press, New York, 1987

Rubright R, MacDonald D: Marketing Health & Human Services. Aspen Publications, Queenstown, Maryland, 1981

Sachs L: Do-It-Yourself Marketing For The Professional Practice. Prentice-Hall, New Jersey, 1986

Trei EW (ed): Public Relations Workbook. Private Practice Section—APTA, Alexandria, VA, 1983

APPENDIX 10-1

Sample Marketing Plan

NAME OF COMPANY X
MARKETING PLAN

I. Background of Company

Company X is a private practice outpatient facility owned and operated by four physical therapists. It is located in Anytown, U.S.A., and was established in 1990.

  A. Mission Statement

    To provide community-based physical therapy services to individuals with various types of medical and physical disabilities to assist them in achieving a maximum level of functioning.

    Company X will provide intensive physical therapy treatment to all its patients. The patient, the patient's family and "significant others" will be encouraged to participate in the treatment whenever appropriate.

    Company X will be fully equipped to provide quality treatment to its patients.

  B. Description of Services

    Specialized programs will be developed as a result of community needs. Currently Company X provides evaluation and treatment of patients with the following problems:

    1. Back and neck dysfunction
    2. Orthopedics and sports injuries
    3. Hand injuries
    4. Rheumatologic problems
    5. Open wounds/burns
    6. Neurologic problems

II. Situational analysis

  A. Market Area

    1. Primary Service Area—Majority Town, U.S.A. (the area where the majority of the patients reside). It can consist of several zip code areas, a county, part of a county, city, town, etc.

    2. Secondary Service Area—where the minority of the patients reside.

  B. Population Trends

    The population of the primary service area is significantly older, with a slightly higher than average median income ($23,212). 24 percent of the population is age 65 and older. 21 percent is female between ages 15 and 44. In 1988 the population was 702,967; it is expected to increase to 842,988 by 1992 (a 19.1 percent increase).

C. Cultural/Social Conditions

Although the population majority is slightly older, the influx of new businesses and migration from other states is bringing a large number of young adults to the area.

D. Key Industries

There are 18,120 businesses operating in the primary and secondary service areas, employing over 250,000 people. Approximately 35 percent of these firms are involved with providing services and 30.2 percent are involved with retail trade. A major employer is Company A, with 10,500 employees. Other light industry employers are Companies B, C, and D.

E. Schools

In the primary service area, there are three elementary schools, four junior high schools, five high schools, three alternative education schools and one adult education school.

F. Health Care Providers

1. *Acute Care Hospitals*—There are three acute care hospitals in the primary service area and eight in the secondary service area. Two of the acute care hospitals are proprietary and one is a not-for-profit hospital in the primary service area. Fifty percent of the secondary service area hospitals are proprietary.

2. *Physicians*—The total number of physicians in the primary service area is 724. There is a large pool of potential referral sources.

3. *Physical Therapists*—There are four physical therapist-owned private practices and seven physician-owned physical therapy settings.

4. *Chiropractors*—There are 28 chiropractors in the primary service area; about three-fourths of them provide their own therapy services; the other one-fourth refer to physical therapists.

III. Environmental/Political Issues Affecting the Practice

A. A large teaching hospital is located across the street from the company and has an established physical therapy outpatient practice and referral patterns.

B. Although current physician practices are relatively unaffected by health maintenance organizations (HMOs) and preferred provider organizations (PPOs), many physicians (particularly internists and general practitioners) fear erosion of their practices; thus, there is increasing interest in joint ventures and marketing.

IV. Self-perceived Strengths and Weaknesses

A. Strengths

1. Excellent programs

2. High quality, positive staff

    3. Motivated owners
    4. Good marketing skills and contacts
    5. No aides—licensed professional therapists only
    6. Good location—across the street from an acute care hospital
  B. Weaknesses
    1. No brochure
    2. Seven physician-owned physical therapist settings in primary service area
    3. Physician allegiance to local hospitals
    4. $500 cap on Medicare Part B
    5. Large Medicare population

V. Marketing Goals
    1. Increase average weekly outpatient visits from 150 to 300 by the end of the next fiscal year.
    2. Change the payer mix from 50 percent Medicare, 25 percent Workers' Compensation, and 25 percent private insurance to 35 percent Medicare, 25 percent Workers' Compensation, and 40 percent private insurance by the end of the next fiscal year.
    3. Develop a Speaker's Bureau by July 15, 19–– and schedule at least two speaking engagements per month.
    4. Send out at least one press release per month to all area newspapers.
    5. Join the local Mayor's Committee for the Disabled by July 1, 19–– and participate in the scheduled meetings.
    6. Participate weekly in the Arthritis Aquasize Program.
    7. Meet with at least two physicians per week during fiscal year 19––.
    8. Visit at least three industries per month during fiscal year 19–– to obtain referrals.
    9. Negotiate contracts with all HMOs in the area by October 15, 19––.
  10. Visit with at least two rehabilitation specialists or outside agencies per week.
  11. Hold an office manager's luncheon on September 21, 19–– to help generate referrals.
  12. Develop a brochure by July 1, 19–– to use when making direct sales calls and for doing direct mailouts.
  13. Do at least one direct mailout per month to the target market or sub-markets.

VI. Target Market and Sub-markets
The broad target market is anyone needing physical therapy services. Some marketing planners would segment or divide the target market to reach one or more similar groups of people. Then they would plan a separate marketing mix strategy for each. However, this approach is better used in the manufacturing industries. For physical therapists, the combined target market approach, which merges many sub-markets into one big target market, can be used. The submarkets include anyone who can make a direct or indirect referral to the private practice (see Ch. 11).

VII. Tracking Forms

A tracking form is a record that keeps (at a minimum) data on dates and times of marketing contacts, who was involved, the results of the contact, and the follow-up plans. The marketing report form in Appendix 10-2 is a sample of what could be done on a weekly basis. The person filling out the report may do it as follows:

1. *Name*—the person, program or specialty area that has made the contacts
2. *Date and Time*—when the marketing contact was made
3. *Contact/Company*—the specific person contacted along with the name of the company, agency, or group to which this person belongs. The contact can be written, by phone, or by personal contact
4. *Staff Involved*—the names of any personnel involved
5. *Plan*—a specific plan such as "sign contract" or general plan such as "generate referrals"
6. *Outcome*—basically indicates what happened, e.g., "contract signed" or "received two referrals"
7. *Other Marketing Activities*—any other activities that were performed that the marketer does not wish to forget: direct mailout descriptions, a vendor meeting about a "giveaway," etc

Another type of tracking form is the referral log, which provides an area to record referrals by referral source, i.e., physician, agency, etc. This form can be customized to suit the individual practice. The data will keep the administrator aware of any growth, decrease, or leveling off of the number of referrals from a particular source. It also allows the tracking of diagnoses, outcomes, and the length of time it has been since a patient of a particular physician was seen. Computerization utilizing a data-base system would be the most efficient method of tallying and manipulating the data to provide information to the marketing and administrative personnel and should be used if available.

APPENDIX 10-2

MARKETING REPORT

NAME _____

Date and Time	Contact/ Company	Staff Involved	Plan	Outcome

Other Marketing Date	Contact/ Company	Activity	Plan	Outcome
1.				
2.				
3.				
4.				
5.				
6.				
7.				
8.				
9.				

11

REFERRAL SOURCES

The importance of creating a marketing strategy to promote the new private physical therapy practice is discussed in Chapter 10. This chapter briefly discusses the many referral sources that can be used in the marketing effort and concludes with a discussion of *direct access* for physical therapists (i.e., provision of patient care by physical therapists without formal referral from physicians).

When soliciting referrals from any potential source, physical therapists should always emphasize what they can do for the referral source. For example, the practice's ability to refer patients to the physician would be an asset to the referral source. In appealing to potential referral sources, it is important to stress the attributes that work best for one's own practice. A strong, athletic man projects a certain image, an energetic, verbally gifted woman another. A physical therapist with advanced academic credentials can use these as a selling point, whereas a physical therapist with only a bachelor's degree cannot. Therefore, physical therapists must identify the attributes that work to their advantage when appealing to potential referral sources.

PHYSICIANS

There are many different specialties within the medical profession, each providing care to patients with many different diseases or dysfunctions. Therefore, a medical specialist's need to refer patients to other physician specialists or to physical therapists will vary according to the chosen specialty. Each medical specialist treats different patient populations, many of whom would benefit from procedures offered by a physical therapist. This provides physical therapy private practitioners with different avenues to pursue when trying to secure medical referrals.

When appealing to physicians and all potential sources for referrals, one must stress the assets of the private practice, which may include location, fees, hours of operation, and, most importantly, unique clinical attributes.

Orthopedic Surgeons

Since orthopedic surgeons treat musculoskeletal dysfunctions, they are inherently the largest medical source of referrals to physical therapy. However, even within orthopedic medicine there are subspecialties, such as sports medicine, joint replacements, spinal dysfunction, and hand surgery. When approaching orthopedic surgeons for referrals, the practice's equipment and clinical skills should be emphasized. If the practice owns specialty equipment such as isokinetic machines, whirlpools, and biofeedback units, this may be the key to convincing the orthopedist. When explaining how the private practice meets the needs of the orthopedic surgeon's specialty areas, the physical therapist should relate these needs to the clinical skills and the available equipment that would most likely be used.

Neurologists

Neurologists provide care to patients with neurologic dysfunctions. Within this framework there are three types of patient problems that frequently require physical therapy services: central nervous system disorders, spinal dysfunctions that may irritate or compress nerve roots, and peripheral nerve dysfunctions. When soliciting neurologists the physical therapist should stress the practice's equipment and clinical skills and should discuss which of the three types of dysfunctions the practice desires to treat. The therapist's relevant advanced credentials, such as neurodevelopmental treatment (NDT) certification in treating neurologic patients should be pointed out.

Neurosurgeons

Neurosurgeons work in conjunction with orthopedic surgeons and neurologists. Some neurosurgeons primarily operate on patients with spinal dysfunctions, whereas others perform surgery for problems relating to the central nervous system. Whatever patient population they may treat, their patients usually require physical therapy. When soliciting referrals from neurosurgeons, physical therapists should realize that postsurgical rehabilitation may be their strongest selling point.

Rheumatologists

Rheumatologists work primarily with arthritic patients, a population frequently made up largely of older people, who are apt to have osteoarthritic changes, leading to complaints of pain that are frequently associated with the spine and extremity joints. Arthritic populations also have diseases classified as rheumatologic disorders, which span all age groups. Rheumatologists frequently use medications, including those given by injection, as part of their treatment. It is up to the physical therapist in private practice to educate rheumatologists about how physical therapy can assist patients with arthritic problems. The use of transcutaneous electrical nerve stimulation (TENS) units for pain management and of ultrasound and iontophoresis to complement injections are a few examples.

Plastic Surgeons

Plastic surgeons treat a large variety of patients, some of whom require physical therapy. For example, patients who have undergone surgery for traumatic hand injuries require rehabilitation, as do patients with wounds that require whirlpool treatment and dressing changes. Even patients who have undergone liposuction procedures may benefit from postsurgical ultrasound treatments. Once again, educating plastic surgeons about what the practice offers their patients may prove valuable.

Family Practitioners

Family practitioners see patients with all types of diseases and dysfunctions. They frequently refer special problems to physician specialists rather than physical therapists, as usually they are unaware of the benefits of physical therapy. The major thrust in approaching family practitioners is educational; referrals will hopefully follow this education. The major benefit that family practitioners gain from referring patients for physical therapy is that they are less likely to lose patients to the specialist. The lower fees for physical therapy constitute another selling point. Family practitioners must be convinced that the physical therapist will request intervention by a medical specialist when necessary.

Internists

Physicians who specialize in internal medicine are very similar to family practitioners, since they see patients with all types of diseases and dysfunctions. In addition, many internists also have a specialty area, such as rheumatology, cardiology, or oncology. The major emphasis in soliciting these physicians is education. In addition to using a strategy similar to that used with family practitioners, the benefits of physical therapy for the internist's specialty area should be emphasized.

Emergency Medicine Physicians

The horizons of emergency medicine physicians have broadened. They now practice in two different settings: the conventional hospital emergency room and a newer type of setting, the 24-hour emergency center. Walk-in cases are treated in both environments. Hospital-based emergency room physicians primarily treat emergencies whereas emergency center physicians also serve as family practitioners. Both types of physicians lack education about physical therapy services and need to be made aware of conditions in which physical therapy would prove helpful. Emergency room physicians are accustomed to referring to physician specialists, so this habit will take time to change.

Physiatrists

Physiatrists are experts in physical medicine and rehabilitation, and as such they do not require education about physical therapy; their patients require physical therapy or related services primarily. Since most physiatrists are hospital employees and generally oversee the rehabilitation services, they refer mainly within the hospital. The marketing approach to physiatrists would be to highlight those services provided by the private practice but not by the hospital.

Cardiologists

Cardiologists are experts on the physiology and diseases of the heart. Those who believe in the benefits of therapeutic exercise have two types of patients who can use physical therapy. One is the physically unfit person with hypertension, who may require a medication regimen, a special diet, and a monitored physical exercise program. The second type is the patient who is undergoing cardiac rehabilitation following heart surgery. A general private physical therapy practice is capable of providing the later stages of a cardiac rehabilitation program. For both types of patients the physical therapy practice would require equipment for aerobic conditioning and qualified personnel to monitor the patient's vital signs.

Vascular Surgeons

Vascular surgeons deal with problems ranging from minor vascular conditions to those requiring bypasses and amputations. Rehabilitation for these patients may include hygiene for impaired circulation, wound management, fitness programs, and training that precedes or accompanies use of a prosthesis. Informing vascular surgeons that the practice has an interest in such patients may generate referrals.

Pulmonary Physicians

Pulmonary physicians deal with respiratory diseases or dysfunctions, ranging from mild asthma to removal of a lung. Rehabilitation for their patients may include instruction in proper breathing techniques, postural drainage, and generalized conditioning exercises. Educating pulmonary physicians that the practice has an interest in such patients may prove beneficial.

Thoracic Surgeons

Thoracic surgeons deal with patients who require thoracic surgery for many diverse reasons. Regardless of the procedure, such surgery is extremely invasive and has an adverse impact on the patient's ability to breathe naturally, efficiently, and without pain. For these patients physical therapy can provide a rehabilitation program similar to that for pulmonary patients. Informing thoracic surgeons that the practice has an interest in such patients may generate referrals.

Obstetricians

Obstetricians may be referral sources since women frequently develop low back dysfunction and other musculoskeletal problems during pregnancy. Physical therapists are able to provide relief for many pregnant women with low back pain, but obstetricians are usually not familiar with the services provided by physical therapists. Therefore, when appealing to them, education is critical. Moreover, since it is essential that physical therapists emphasize the safety of mother and child, they should discuss with the obstetrician which physical therapy procedures are indicated and which are contraindicated.

Pediatricians

Pediatricians are potential referral sources, since children may develop a multitude of problems, including fractures, scoliosis, and neurologic problems, all of which may require physical therapy. However, pediatricians usually refer specific problems to physicians who specialize in the respective areas. When appealing to pediatricians, physical therapists should emphasize their educational backgrounds.

Oncologists

Oncologists provide care to patients with problems associated with cancer. These patients may have a multitude of problems. Cancer patients who would benefit from physical therapy services are postsurgical patients, in whom physical therapy rehabilitation may decrease pain, enhance range of motion, improve strength, and improve respiratory abilities. As in dealing with other physicians, the physical therapist's educational background should be emphasized.

Head and Neck Physicians

Head and neck physicians provide care to patients with problems ranging from posttraumatic reconstruction (also treated by plastic surgeons) to cancer of the head and neck region (also treated by oncologists). Educating head and neck physicians to the merits of physical therapy services may generate patient referrals.

Psychiatrists

Psychiatrists provide medical and psychological care for patients with psychological problems or disorders, which frequently are related to drug abuse, chronic pain, and stress. Physical therapy services can assist psychiatrists in rehabilitating patients with such problems or disorders by offering fitness programs, pain management, and stress reduction programs as adjunct treatments. Since psychiatrists are usually not familiar with the benefits of physical therapy for their patients, educating them in this area may open up a new avenue of patient referrals.

NONMEDICAL DOCTORS

Oral Surgeons

Oral surgeons provide medical and surgical intervention for patients with mouth-related problems. Temporomandibular joint dysfunction is one disorder frequently managed by the oral surgeon. This condition is associated with problems of the cervical and thoracic spines, as well as with headaches. Coordination of the services of the oral surgeon and the physical therapist is helpful to many patients. Therefore, education of oral surgeons and development of a working relationship with them may open up a new avenue of patient referrals.

Dentists

Dentists, along with oral surgeons, frequently treat patients with temporomandibular joint dysfunction. Coordination of the services of the dentist, oral surgeon, and physical therapist makes for a most effective treatment team. Therefore, education of dentists and development of a working relationship with them may open up a new avenue of patient referrals.

Podiatrists

Podiatrists treat foot problems both by conservative management and by surgery. Physical therapy frequently provides rehabilitation for their patients. Therefore, a natural working relationship should exist between podiatrists and physical therapists.

Chiropractors

Chiropractors treat patients with problems of spinal origin; however, they rarely emphasize muscle strength, muscle flexibility, and overall fitness. In addition, chiropractors frequently have patients who complain of extremity dysfunctions. Therefore, physical therapy, which does emphasize muscle strength, muscle flexibility, and overall fitness should be the natural complement to chiropractic care. To cultivate referrals from chiropractors, physical therapists must emphasize the complementary rather than the common procedures that their practice offers.

Veterinarians

The role of physical therapy in the rehabilitation of animals is growing. Physical therapists wishing to work in this area need to have knowledge of animals and interest in working with veterinarians.

HEALTH CARE PROFESSIONALS

Nurses

Nurses can serve as referral sources to physical therapy practices in an indirect or a direct manner. Indirect referrals are made through their many contacts with physicians and patients. Also, nurses are frequently in a position to refer patients directly to physical therapy; for example, a nurse working directly with a physician and implementing the physician's orders becomes the direct referring source if one of the orders is to send a patient to physical therapy. In addition, nurses in charge of home health care agencies refer homebound clients directly to physical therapists.

Occupational Therapists

Occupational therapists, like physical therapists, provide care to patients with many different diseases and disorders. Frequently patients require both types of therapy, in which case the occupational therapist can refer patients to a private physical therapy practice.

Speech Pathologists

Speech pathologists are another group of therapists who provide care to patients who suffer from many different diseases and disorders and who frequently also require physical therapy services. In this case speech pathologists can refer patients to private physical therapy practices.

Respiratory Therapists

Respiratory therapists, like physical therapists, provide care to patients with many different diseases and disorders and when both services are necessary, can refer patients to private physical therapy practices.

Physical Therapists

Physical therapists frequently refer patients to other physical therapists on the basis of geography, specialty skills, office hours, and acceptance of specific insurance reimbursement. Furthermore, hospital physical therapists may refer patients to local private practices when the department has too many patients.

Physician Assistants

Physician assistants work directly with physicians and implement their orders. If one of the orders is to send a patient to physical therapy, the physician assistant becomes the direct referring source.

Psychologists

Psychologists treat patients with psychological problems or disorders, which are frequently related to drug abuse, chronic pain, and stress. Physical therapists can assist psychologists in rehabilitating patients with such problems or disorders by offering fitness programs, pain management, and stress reduction programs as adjunct therapy. Since psychologists are usually not familiar with the benefits of physical therapy for their patients, educating them about the merits of physical therapy services may open up a new avenue of patient referrals.

Social Workers

Social workers provide counseling and vocational advice to individuals and families in need of support because of physical or psychological problems or disorders. Physical therapy services can assist social workers in rehabilitating patients, however, like psychologists, they require education about physical therapy services.

Office Staff

The office staffs of physicians frequently implement the physician's order. If one of the orders is to send a patient to physical therapy, the office staff becomes the direct referring source.

Rehabilitation Specialists

Rehabilitation specialists, frequently called *rehabilitation nurses* or *counselors*, are people who take over the management of patients' cases and coordinate Workers' Compensation or catastrophic illness cases. Rehabilitation specialists usually work for the insurance carrier directly or as independent agents; in fact, they serve as case managers, whose duty is to see that appropriate medical care is provided and costs are controlled. If complete medical recovery is not possible, the rehabilitation specialist will coordinate vocational training, counseling, etc. to maximize the patient's recovery.

Physical Trainers

Physical trainers provide training for people who desire to become physically fit, either in health clubs or individually in the person's home. Physical trainers can develop working relationships with physical therapists by referring to them clients who develop musculoskeletal problems. Therapists can reciprocate by referring to trainers people who are past the musculoskeletal dysfunction stage and need only physical fitness training.

OTHER SOURCES
Insurance Carriers

Insurance carriers are concerned about the high cost of medically related health care. If the practice can document quality care at decreased cost, either by charging lower fees or by giving fewer treatments per patient, insurance companies will provide referrals. However, finding a person of authority in an insurance company to listen to the facts may prove difficult.

Health Maintenance Organizations

Health maintenance organizations provide insurance coverage for clients under many restrictions, a primary restriction being that the client must use health care providers who have contracts with the respective health maintenance organization. Physical therapy providers can frequently make such contracts for a set fee or a percentage of the normal fee.

Industries

Industrial concerns pay large medical premiums to provide health insurance for their employees. Therefore they desire to keep their employees healthy and at work and also to provide fast and cost-effective rehabilitation to those who are injured. Physical therapy is able to offer to industry ergonomic modification, preemployment screening, functional capacity evaluations, work hardening, and high-quality rehabilitation. Explaining how the services economically serve the industry is critical. However, it is usually difficult to establish the contact with the people who make decisions about health care, such as the director of personnel, comptroller, risk manager, administrator, employee health nurse, and occupational physician.

Health Care Consumers

The consumers of physical therapy services include both people who presently require and people who do not presently require such services. These consumers are frequently overlooked when marketing physical therapy private practices. Consumers need to feel that the health care provider truly cares for them; both the environment of the private practice and its philosophy of patient care can give the consumer confidence that this is the case. The quality of care provided and the results will also influence the consumer, as will the cost factor. Thus a physical therapy practice, by developing the appropriate philosophy and environment, can solicit the consumer directly, but here also education about what physical therapy is and what it can do is essential. Consumers also need to learn how to obtain a referral to a particular private practice when dealing with referring physicians. The concept of appealing directly to the consumer is essential, as the profession is moving toward direct access.

PERSONAL MARKETING MEETING

Arranging the Meeting

The hardest part of the personal marketing meeting is arranging it. This can be done either by stopping in personally or by telephoning the office of the potential referral source. Whichever method is used, the problem of getting past the front office staff and arranging the meeting can be major. Sometimes front office personnel such as office managers are able to set up the meeting, but at other times office staff must clear the meeting with the potential referral source. These persons usually say that they will call back after speaking with the potential referral source, but frequently they do not call back. In many instances busy people who are potential referral sources give the front office a blanket rule not to arrange meetings.

When visiting or telephoning an office, one must quickly explain the purpose of the call, which is usually to introduce the private practice. It is important to explain that this meeting will take 5 minutes or at most 10. One must sound positive and confident during this initial interaction. If visiting in person, one should immediately present the business card and should always have promotional literature available. If a meeting cannot be arranged, it is a good idea to leave some promotional literature about the practice. When telephone calls do not result in an appointment, the front office staff should at least be informed that an introductory letter will follow. The letter should then be sent and should include promotional literature.

The Meeting

The personal marketing meeting is very valuable. The personal, face-to-face contact increases the potential for referrals. If the referral source knows the physical therapist personally, even if for only a few minutes, this is likely to have some effect. When personally approaching physicians, one should realize they are very busy. Physical therapists will usually be allotted about 5 minutes to market their practice, but occasionally a lunch meeting with a potential referral source can be arranged, which will increase the likelihood of the physical therapist and the potential referral source coming to know each other. Regardless of the length of the meeting, the positive and unique aspects of the practice should be emphasized. Some of these features may be ownership by physical therapists, the fact that only licensed therapists provide patient care, special equipment, the fee for service, and extended office hours. One should try not to speak derogatorily about other physical therapy providers in the community. It may prove helpful to know the physician's physical therapy referral pattern before the meeting so that the meeting may be so conducted as to maximize patient referrals. Before concluding the meeting, the physical therapist should ask about the potential referring physician's preference in type of patients treated and should request business cards in the event that the therapist has patients to refer to the physician.

DIRECT ACCESS

Direct access denotes the stature the physical therapy profession has achieved and the progress it has made in the eyes of consumers, health professionals, and legislatures. *Direct access* is the term used to describe the situation in which consumers can go directly to physical therapists and receive services without being medically referred for treatment.

The physical therapy profession through the years has been prescription- or referral-driven, which means that for patients to receive physical therapy, they must be referred to the physical therapy provider. This obviously places physical therapists in a subordinate position with respect to referring physicians. In addition, this system makes it harder for consumers to make contact with physical therapists and increases the cost of medical care.

Starting in the early 1970s the American Physical Therapy Association began investigating the possibility of physical therapists becoming direct access providers. Eventually the association endorsed this concept provided it was permitted under state law. The next step was to prevail upon states not allowing direct access to modify their laws governing physical therapy practice. This campaign has been carried on by the American Physical Therapy Association's State chapters in the affected states. In 21 states legislation has been enacted to allow direct access to physical therapists (Table 11-1), and 40 states (including these 21) have at least a modified form of direct access, allowing physical therapists to evaluate patients without a physician's referral (Table 11-2). The legislative battle continues in the states that do not have direct access.

The importance of direct access legislation is obvious to private practitioners, since it allows physical therapy practitioners to market their service directly to the consumer. As a result physical therapy is in a better position to compete in the health care marketplace.

Table 11-1. States with Direct Access (1989)

Alaska	Kentucky	New Hampshire
Arizona	Maryland	North Dakota
California	Massachusetts	South Dakota
Colorado	Minnesota	Utah
Idaho	Montana	Vermont
Illinois	Nebraska	Washington
Iowa	Nevada	West Virginia

Table 11-2. States with a Modified Form of Direct Access (1989)

Alaska	Maine	North Carolina
Arizona	Maryland	North Dakota
California	Massachusetts	Oklahoma
Colorado	Michigan	Pennsylvania
Connecticut	Minnesota	Rhode Island
Florida	Mississippi	South Dakota
Georgia	Montana	Tennessee
Hawaii	Nebraska	Texas
Idaho	Nevada	Utah
Illinois	New Hampshire	Vermont
Iowa	New Jersey	Washington
Kansas	New Mexico	West Virginia
Kentucky	New York	Wyoming
Louisiana		

SUMMARY

This chapter discusses the many possible referral sources available to the physical therapist in private practice. Suggestions on what to emphasize when soliciting the various possible referral sources have been included. Additionally, direct solicitation of the consumer of physical therapy services is addressed, along with the implications of direct access.

SUGGESTED READINGS

American Physical Therapy Association, Division of Professional Relations: Direct Access To Physical Therapy. American Physical Therapy Association, Alexandria, VA, 1987

Fiebert I, Rohan J, Wise H, Parry K: Communicating with physicians. Clin Management 3(1):26–27, Winter 1983

Kaplan EA: Using public relations to support direct access campaigns. Phys Ther Today 11(1):30–31, Spring 1988

Profile of a private practice physical therapist—results of the PPS survey. Whirlpool 8(2):26–29, Summer 1985

12

REIMBURSEMENT AND OFFICE MANAGEMENT

In the health care delivery system, the traditional fee-for-service method of payment is changing drastically. Trends affecting the reimbursement of physical therapy services include

1. Diverging arrangements for payment and collection through contracts with third-party payers
2. Medicare regulations that include capitation and a percentage discount
3. Increasing utilization of services by Health Maintenance Organizations (HMOs) and Preferred Provider Organizations (PPOs)
4. Patient awareness and concern regarding the cost of services
5. Workers' Compensation programs in the respective states clamping down on abuse of the programs by both patient and providers.

The changing dynamics of the health care system significantly affect the accounting/billing system. Being adaptable and staying on top of current reimbursement issues are essential.

Although the office staff will be responsible for the implementation of the billing system, final responsibility remains with the private practitioner. Physical therapists receive little education in physical therapy programs in the art and process of office management. The art is learned by trial and error and on–the–spot training. This method of learning is costly in the private practice setting.

This chapter discusses the practical aspects of establishing a billing and accounting system. Sample forms and letters are provided for future use.

MAJOR THIRD PARTY PAYERS
Blue Cross/Blue Shield

Blue Cross/Blue Shield plans, organized as not-for-profit corporations, pride themselves on maintaining a low administrative overhead. Blue Cross plans, service plans that pay for hospitalization costs, pay the hospitals directly under a contract.

Blue Shield plans, service plans that pay for physician and other provider costs, pay the providers by a standard fee schedule. The practice must file an application to receive a provider number. *Participating providers* accept the fee schedule as payment in full. *Nonparticipating providers* do not accept the Blue Shield payment as payment in full. The patient is responsible for the difference between the fee schedule and the provider's bill.

Medicare

Medicare is a federally sponsored program administered by the Health Care Financing Administration (HCFA). Medicare, part of the Social Security system, is provided for in Title XVIII of the Social Security Act. It is designed to help patients meet their medical expenses upon reaching the age of 65. Medicare pays only about 40 percent of total health care expenditures.

There are two parts to Medicare: Part A, a compulsory program, and Part B, a voluntary program. Under Part A (Hospital Insurance), benefits are paid for hospital care, care provided in extended-care facilities, and certain types of follow-up care. Part B (Supplementary Medical Insurance) covers the care provided by physicians, whether incurred at the office, home, or hospital. In addition, it pays for certain related services, such as physical therapy and diagnostic tests. Part B is optional medical insurance, for which the patient pays a monthly premium. The two parts of Medicare work together to provide a single broad-based insurance program.

Private insurance organizations, known as intermediaries or carriers, handle Medicare payments under contract to the federal government. Under Part A, each institution for health care makes its own selection of the intermediary. Under Part B of the program, HCFA assigns an intermediary in each state. Appendix 12-1 provides a list of names and addresses of state intermediaries.

Becoming a Medicare Provider

Outpatient physical therapy is a service covered under Part B of the Medicare program when the service is furnished by or under arrangements with a qualified provider or facility. An approved facility or provider is one that meets all state and local licensing requirements and passes the certification requirements set by the HCFA.

In private practice, there are four available options to consider regarding Medicare:

1. Do not accept Medicare
2. Apply for independent practitioner status not accepting assignment
3. Apply for independent practitioner status accepting assignment
4. Apply to become a Medicare-certified rehabilitation agency.

Option 1

If the practice does not accept Medicare patients, it means that the practice was never inspected by a Medicare representative. The practice has decided not to accept the terms of the Medicare system and Medicare patients treated by the practice will not receive reimbursement from Medicare.

Option 2

The practitioner applies for Medicare approval as an independent practitioner. A physical therapist is considered to be in independent practice specifically if the therapist renders services free of the administrative and professional control of an employer such as a physician, institution, or agency; the patients treated are the therapist's own patients; and the therapist has the right to collect fees for the services rendered.

Once recognized as an independent practitioner under the Medicare program, the practitioner must follow Medicare reimbursement regulations whether the practice is a participating or nonparticipating provider:

1. The patient is only covered for the first $500 of physical therapy during each calendar year.
2. The patient is responsible for paying the 20 percent copayment and the $75 annual deductible.
3. Only the physical therapist with the Medicare provider number is allowed to treat the patient.
4. Physical therapists who do not participate may accept assignment at their discretion.

Option 3

Additional regulations apply if the decision to participate has been made. The major additional regulations that apply are

1. Participation means that assignment of the charges is accepted and that the practice may not collect from the beneficiary more than the applicable deductible and coinsurance for covered services when assignment is accepted.
2. The Medicare intermediary is responsible for generating payment on clean claims within a shorter period of time and the payment is made directly to the provider.
3. Assignment must be accepted on all Medicare claims.
4. The practice submits the claim directly to Medicare rather than to the patient.

Option 4

Under the Medicare program, the process to become a certified rehabilitation agency is lengthy. However, if the decision to go this route is made, the following reimbursement regulations apply:

1. Medicare Part B intermediaries are responsible for making payments on a reasonable-cost basis to participating clinic providers.
2. The principles of reimbursement applicable to hospitals, skilled nursing facilities, and home health agencies that participate in the Medicare Program also are applicable to providers of outpatient physical therapy services.

Accepting Assignment

Accepting Medicare assignment means that (1) the practice will bill Medicare and receive direct payments for services rendered; (2) the practice will accept Medicare's approved charges for the services provided. The patient is then responsible for 20 percent of the allowable charges and an annual $75 deductible. Assignment may be accepted at the discretion of the provider or for all cases by becoming a participating provider.

Medicare provides a contract, renewable annually, to a participating provider. To encourage providers to participate in the program, Medicare guarantees the provider faster payment and lists the facility in its provider directory.

Factors to consider when deciding to participate are

1. The importance of Medicare patients to the practice
2. The percentage of the practice's patients covered by Medicare
3. The percentage of collection problems that are Medicare claims
4. The loss of patients to participating therapists
5. The disparity between the practice's standard fee schedule and the Medicare allowable fees
6. The number of participating physicians who will still refer to the practice

Regardless of which option the practitioner takes, Medicare seems to do whatever it can to delay payments. For example, in November 1988, HCFA passed a ruling requiring intermediaries to send an information questionnaire to all beneficiaries with pending claims. The intent was to ascertain whether Medicare was the primary or secondary provider for each patient. The beneficiary was requested to complete the questionnaire within 30 days. If there was no response, a second letter was sent. If there was no reply within 45 days, the provider would not be paid for services rendered. The provider was not allowed to provide the beneficiary with the questionnaire when the patient first appeared for treatment. Although the intent of this rule seemed harmless enough, payment was delayed or denied, with the provider having no recourse but to be patient.

Identifying Medicare Recipients

All Medicare recipients will have a red, white, and blue Medicare card. The card will identify Part B recipients with a B after the patient's Social Security number. If an A is after the patient's Social Security number, the recipient is only eligible for Part A benefits. The card also gives the date on which the patient became eligible for benefits, usually the first day of the month in which he or she turned 65 years old. Information regarding whether the patient has met the deductible will only be given to the beneficiary. The intermediary will not give information directly to the provider.

The practitioner must determine whether Medicare is the primary or secondary insurance carrier. The recipients must be asked about other insurance coverage and the circumstances of their injury. If a Medicare patient is still employed and has group medical benefits from his or her employer, Medicare becomes the secondary payer. Furthermore, if the patient sustained the injury in an automobile accident and either driver's auto insurance covers the treatment, Medicare becomes the secondary payer.

Medicare Supplemental Policies

Many insurance companies provide supplemental or secondary policies to fill the gaps that Medicare leaves. These policies are not government sponsored or government approved. Most supplemental policies reimburse the patient only for those services that Medicare allows.

WORKERS' COMPENSATION

Workers' Compensation has been established by law in all states to deal with occupational accidents and diseases occurring at the workplace or in the course of doing one's job. Individual state laws differ regarding actual benefits and reimbursement issues. The practitioner should contact the Workers' Compensation office in the state where the practice will open to find out the state laws (Appendix 12-2). Payment for medical care is made on a fee-for-service basis or with specific limitations regarding a specified maximum amount or limited time period. States differ regarding the selection of the physician who will treat the worker. In some states the worker does not have first choice; the decision regarding physician selection rests with the employer or the insurer.

HEALTH MAINTENANCE ORGANIZATIONS

The HMO is an alternative type of delivery system based on a different philosophy about health services. It stresses preventive measures rather than the acute treatment emphasized by conventional third-party coverages. HMOs provide incentives to the insured and the provider to minimize use of expensive inpatient treatment. Physicians are usually salaried, and beneficiaries pay a fixed fee.

Formal application and contract negotiations between the practice and the HMO occur to determine the fee schedule. Many HMOs have a predetermined reimbursement rate while others will negotiate with individual practices regarding fee schedules. The fee is generally fixed per visit rather than per procedure. Additionally, the patient is referred to the therapist by a primary care physician with a predetermined amount of allowed visits.

PREFERRED PROVIDER ORGANIZATIONS

A relatively new form of health plan receiving increased attention from both payers and providers is the *preferred provider organization*. The number of PPOs is growing in response to a highly competitive health care market. In a PPO, the third-party payer is often a self-insured company or union trust fund that contracts with hospitals, doctors, and others to provide medical services to its constituents. The providers discount prices of services and establish utilization review programs to control costs. In return, the PPO provides prompt payment and a certain volume of patients. If PPO beneficiaries select a nonaffiliated provider, they pay coinsurance and deductibles. If they choose a PPO provider, they receive first-dollar coverage.

PPOs, like HMOs, negotiate contracts with each applicant. The practitioner's proposed fee is generally a discounted percentage of the office's standard fee schedule. Generally, the patient is not referred to the practice with predetermined allowable visits but rather with an ordinary prescription.

ELEMENTS OF COLLECTING MONEY
Establish Fees

A precise accounting of the costs of providing services, including a reasonable profit margin, is consistent with good business practice. It is important to make sure that the fee schedule is simple enough for the patient to understand. The following items must be considered when establishing fees:

1. The *cost* of providing the service
2. The *value* of the service
3. The *competition* or prevailing community rates

Several methods are available to determine cost. One method to use is as follows:

1. Determine revenue-producing hours per month for each therapist. A good estimate is taking $6\frac{1}{2}$ hours/day multiplied by 22 days/month.
2. Determine the breakeven point by dividing monthly expenses by revenue-producing hours.

$$\text{Breakeven} = \frac{\text{Monthly Expenses}}{\text{Revenue hours} \times \text{number of therapists}}$$

$$\text{Breakeven} = \frac{\$5000}{143 \text{ hrs} \times 2 \text{ therapists}} = \$34.96/\text{hour}$$

3. Determine the profit margin expected.

$$\text{Profit} = \$34.96 \times 150\% = \$52.45 \text{ collected revenues/hour of operation}$$

4. Determine whether the intended profit margin rate meets the value criteria and is competitive.

Value is defined as the worth of a service at a certain time and in a given location. Patients are willing to pay a fair fee for good service as long as they value the service.

Knowledge of the competition and its effect on the practice is indispensable in the development of a competent fee schedule. Health services are as price-oriented as other industries. Health services compete in service quality, reputation, location, accessibility, waiting and treatment time, staff availability, attitude, promotional tools, billing policies, and price.

The competitive environment may irreversibly affect the fee schedule. When major changes occur in the local physical therapy community or on an annual basis, the fee schedule must be reviewed. Survival may dictate that the fee schedule be adjusted so that it leaves a profit margin that is less than anticipated in the original business plan. The decreased profit margin will impede the anticipated growth curve.

Establish Billing Policies

Standard guidelines must be developed regarding all fee and billing issues. The professional, not the office staff, must establish the billing guidelines and educate the office staff regarding them. Special situations that arise include professional courtesy, patients unable to pay, installment payments, reduction of fees, and favors asked by referral sources.

Professional courtesy is a tradition within the medical community. The professional obligation is to treat other professionals and their families at a reduced cost. The practice's owners must determine whether the tradition applies to their practice setting and what the percentage reduction will be.

Reduction of fees and providing certain services at no charge come up routinely. Patients have individual requests based on their unique needs. A typical example is the Medicare patient who insists that the office waive the Medicare 20 percent copayment.

Make Financial Arrangements with the Patient

The first question a patient asks when entering the office regards billing. Many offices market that they "bill most third party payers" as a service to the patient. Mature and established practices refuse to bill the insurance companies and expect payment upon services rendered. In either case, the actions of the office staff must be consistent with the billing policies.

Taking the time to educate the consumer regarding billing will increase patient collections. Patients must clearly understand what is expected from them. This is the most important step of making financial arrangements.

The office staff and, in special cases, the physical therapist, must provide the necessary information to the patient. The old school of thought that the professional provider should not discuss financial arrangements with the patient is becoming obsolete. The most effective person to articulate difficult situations is the professional.

An alternative to verbal communication is the provision of written explanations regarding each method of payment. Figure 12-1 illustrates an Explanation of Medicare Billing form developed by an independent private practice. It is given to all Medicare patients when they enter the office. Patients read this before their first treatment. The office staff handles any questions that arise.

Medicare
Billing and Payment Information

Physical Therapy Institute, Inc. has been inspected and certified to treat Medicare recipients. We *do accept assignment.* This means that we agree to accept the fee schedule set by Medicare *and* that we collect the 20% copayment from the patient. In addition, the regulations set by Medicare state that there is a *$500* annual limit for outpatient physical therapy provided by independent private practitioners.

Under the regulation of Part B, *you* are responsible for the following:

1. Providing a written referral from your doctor

2. The first $75 of covered medical services in any calendar year

3. A copayment of 20% of the allowable charge (on a $50 visit you would be responsible for $10)

4. Any fees beyond the $500 annual limit ($500 averages to approximately 9–11 visits).

We, at Physical Therapy Institute, are responsible for the following Medicare billing:

1. Directly bill Medicare up to $500

2. Collect your 20% copayment on a weekly basis and provide you with a receipt

3. Inform you one visit prior to your reaching the $500 annual limit

4. Provide you with any copies of bills you need to submit to your secondary insurance company, free of charge. We *do not* bill secondary carriers.

If you should have any questions regarding your Medicare bills, please feel free to ask Penny, Tillie, or Debbie.

If you require special arrangements beyond your $500 limit, please speak to your individual therapist.

PATIENT SIGNATURE: _____   **DATE** _____

Fig. 12-1. Form explaining Medicare billing.

INSURANCE BENEFITS VERIFICATION

Date: _____

Insured: _____

Insurance Company: _____

Reponding Clerk: _____

****

This confirms my recent conversation with your insurance company regarding your specific insurance coverage. Your coverage has a _____ deductible for accidental injury and a _____ deductible due to sickness, both per calendar year.

Upon satisfying the deductible, the next _____ of eligible expenses are covered at _____ percent.

The following items are specific to your insurance company:

1. _____

2. _____

3. _____

If you have any questions about the above information or any uncertainty regarding insurance coverage, PLEASE don't hesitate to ask us. We are here to help you.

Yes, I have read and understand the above.

_____ _____
SIGNATURE   DATE

Sincerely,

Fig. 12-2. Form for verification of insurance benefits.

Patients are requested to sign the form and are provided with a photocopy of the signed form for their records. This has helped to avoid misunderstandings.

Another procedure that will avoid future misunderstandings with the patient is to provide the patient with a written confirmation of verified insurance benefits (Fig. 12-2). The patient signs this form following verification of insurance benefits by the office staff.

Any procedure that enhances communication between the professional office and the patient aids the collection process. All participating parties must clearly understand their individual responsibilities when financial arrangements are made.

Establish the Method

The decision to bill manually or by computer will have lasting effects. Because this decision will carry over throughout the life of the private practice, it must be made carefully and with a full understanding of each choice. There are strong advantages and disadvantages for each.

Manual/Pegboard

The simplest and least costly billing method is the manual pegboard system, which can provide all of the accounting data needed to manage a small to medium office. Its basic function is to allow the front desk to record charges and receipts simultaneously. There are local and national companies that specialize in setting up manual systems for professional offices. A company should be chosen whose representatives will educate staff in the practice's office and provide support.

Individual patient ledger cards must be set up to enter manually the patient's daily charges and payments. Smaller offices will then photocopy the cards, which will serve as monthly statements. Entries from the patient ledger cards must be posted on a daysheet, which is a daily log of charges, payments, and adjustments for every patient seen and each patient record processed. Meticulous entries, including patient account adjustments, result in an accurate accounts receivable total.

The drawback of this simple and inexpensive method of handling billing is its inefficiency. It takes time and some mathematical prowess to keep the general ledger cards and daysheets up to date. However, if the practice is projected to remain a low-volume office, a manual system is a viable choice.

A manual system is not a viable alternative if the practice is projected to grow into a multitherapist practice that wishes to bill weekly or bi-weekly. It should be considered a first step in setting up a billing system, but if there is a strong sense that computerization will be necessary soon, the money should be spent up front for a computer system. The time required to retroactively enter all the information from your patient records into a computer system is prohibitive.

Computerization

Accounting is the most useful and cost effective function that a computer can accomplish in a medical office. Computerization of the billing system provides the ability to handle increased volume. A well-designed program that prepares the bills, keeps track of delinquent accounts, and breaks down charges by each therapist and cost center saves time.

Completing the standard insurance forms manually is tedious and time-consuming. The patient information portion of the form must be reproduced whenever a manual claim is produced. This wastes time because the patient portion of the insurance claim does not change from billing period to billing period.

The initial process of entering patient information, diagnosis, and insurance information is time-consuming on any computerized billing software programs.

However, once the patient information is entered it never has to be re-entered into the system. The actual visits and modalities/procedures performed during each billing cycle is the only information that needs to be updated. The bills are then produced on insurance forms that feed through the printer. This saves considerable time and effort.

Other advantages of computerization of the billing system include

1. Better follow-up of delinquent accounts
2. Speed of processing
3. Ability to produce increased volume
4. Ready access to patient account information
5. Ability to track productivity of therapists
6. Tracking of physician referrals
7. Access to a spectrum of statistics that assist in practice management
8. Transmitting claims information to insurance carriers electronically rather than by mail

Disadvantages of computerization depend upon the software package purchased. Generic problems include

1. The expense of purchase
2. Dependency on an electronically controlled system that "crashes" sporadically and shuts down when there are power failures
3. Extensive training requirements
4. Dependency on support from the software manufacturer when the billing system has a major problem
5. An annual fee paid to the software company to provide phone support and software updates and enhancements

Outside Company

There are many independent companies in the marketplace that will perform medical billing. Some companies will bring the computer hardware and software in-house and place their trained personnel on site. In-house service may facilitate the process because patient files are on hand for the person entering the data. Other outside services require that the inhouse office staff manually complete information on standardized forms and provide them with daily or weekly charge sheets. The outside service will then perform the billing service at their office. In either situation, the office is charged by entry, by bill produced, or by a contracted monthly fee.

The advantages to having the bills generated by an outside agency are that there is no major capital expense, no direct personnel expense, and the people performing the billing are experts in the field of accounts receivable management. Finally, system failures are the agency's responsibility.

The disadvantages of using an outside agency are that it is more expensive, the patients' records may have to be removed from the office, and the outside agency has no vested interest in getting the bills out in the most timely fashion (they usually have a long-term contract). Additionally, like any other service contract, once signed, the consumer is at the mercy of the billing agency.

Establish the Billing System

Failure to develop an effective billing system can result in large losses of income, increased paperwork, and duplication of effort. Improved cash flow and decreased delinquent accounts will be the major by-products of a well organized billing program.

Billing requirements and procedures are arduous. Procedures must be altered and modified and new ones will constantly emerge. This will assist the office staff in contending with changes in requirements and individual patient requirements.

Steps in Billing

Obtain Information from the Patient

An additional 15 minutes is required to register patients when they are scheduled for their first appointments. When the patient arrives, he or she should be greeted warmly and given an office registration form (Fig. 12-3). The form should be on a clipboard with a pen attached so the patient can sit comfortably in the waiting room while filling out the form. Some patients may require additional assistance from the office staff in completing the form.

An alternative to this method is to interview the patient in a private room for the information. The office staff is then responsible for completing the registration form or entering the information directly into the computer at the time of the interview.

Ask Patient for Insurance Identification Card and Photocopy Both Sides

Regardless of the method used, photocopying all insurance cards and obtaining any special insurance forms will assist in registering the patient. It also avoids mistakes, and the card generally has the insurance company's contract number on it. The practitioner should not rely on the patient's memory or hand-written contract number.

Obtain Signatures and Releases

The patient's signature is required on the claim forms to authorize the release of medical information. In addition, it is required on every claim form submitted when assignment is accepted. The patient does not have to sign each claim form if a signed Lifetime Signature Authorization form is in the patient's file (Fig. 12-4). At the time the claim form is submitted the billing clerk writes "signature on file" in the appropriate box of the claim form.

Patient: _____ Birthdate: _____

Address: _____ City: _____ Zip: _____

Home phone: _____ Work phone: _____

Patient's Soc. Security No.: _____ Insured SS#: _____

Referred by Dr.: _____ Next M.D. Appt.: _____

If Privately Insured:

      Company: _____

      Address: _____

      Telephone: _____

Group Policy No.: _____

If Workers' Compensation:

      Employer: _____

      Address: _____

      Telephone: _____ Injury Date: _____

      Carrier No.: _____

Insurance Co.: _____

      Address: _____

If Automobile Accident:

Insured: _____ Date of Accident: _____

File #: _____ Policy #: _____

Insurance Co. & Local Address: _____

_____

The patient is responsible for all physical therapy fees regardless of insurance coverage. I authorize the release of any medical information necessary to process this claim.

_____
Signature

Fig. 12-3. Patient registration form.

ASSIGNMENT OF INSURANCE BENEFITS

The undersigned hereby authorizes the release of any information relating to all claims for benefits submitted on behalf of myself and/or dependents. I further expressly agree and acknowledge that my signature on this document authorizes my physical therapist to submit claims for benefits for services rendered or for services to be rendered, without obtaining my signature on each and every claim to be submitted for myself and/or dependents, and that I will be bound by this signature as though the undersigned has personally signed the particular claim.

I _____ hereby authorize _____

_____ to pay and hereby assign directly to

Physical Therapy Institute, Inc. all benefits, if any, otherwise payable to me for his/her services as described on the submitted forms.   I understand I am financially responsible for all charges incurred.   I further acknowledge that any insurance benefits, when received by and paid to Physical Therapy Institute, Inc. will be credited to my account, in accordance with the above said agreement.

_____ Date _____
Authorized Signature of Subscriber

Fig. 12-4. Lifetime Signature Authorization form.

Determine Insurance Coverage

While the patient is receiving the first treatment or during the first 24 hours, the information provided by the patient on the registration form must be verified. The receptionist should confirm the insurance coverage by calling the designated insurance company. The insurance company should confirm the amount of the annual deductible and whether the patient has met it. In addition, available benefits for outpatient physical therapy and any specific requirements for the claim form must be discussed. If the patient has more than one insurance plan, the primary insurer must be identified. Request the name of the clerk providing the information in case inconsistencies arise when payment is made.

Assign Appropriate Diagnosis Codes

When a referral is received, whether verbally or in writing, a diagnosis must be provided by the referral source. Office personnel then translate the diagnosis to numbered ICD-9 codes, required by all government programs and by most insurance companies. Every claim submitted for reimbursement and every receipt given to a patient must include the appropriate codes. For proper reimbursement, the office personnel must become very familiar with this coding system. Office personnel must be provided with an ICD-9-CM book and be

PHYSICAL THERAPY STATEMENT

PATIENT'S NAME _____

S. S. NO. _____

INSURED'S NAME _____

INSURED'S ADDRESS _____

REFERRING PHYSICIAN _____

PHYSICAL MEDICINE MODALITIES

97010	Hot or Cold Packs
97012	Traction (Mechanical)
97014	Electrical Stim. (Unattended)
97016	Vasopneumatic Devices
97018	Paraffin Bath
97022	Whirlpool Bath
97039	Unlisted Modality

PHYSICAL MEDICINE PROCEDURES
(Initial 30 minutes)

97110	Therapeutic Ex./Isokinetic
97112	Neuromuscular Re-education
97114	Functional Activities
97116	Gait Training
97118	Electrical Stim. (Manual)
97120	Iontophoresis/Phonophoresis
97122	Traction (Manual)
97124	Massage/Tissue Mobilization
97128	Ultrasound
97139	Unlisted Procedure
97145	Phys. Med. Proc. (ea. add. 15 min.)

97530	Kinetic Act.
97531	Additional 15 Mins.
97520	Prosthetic Training
97500	Orthotic Training-Init. 30 min.
97720	Extremity Testing-Init. 30 min.
97752	Cybex Testing (with Analysis)
99912	Transcutaneous Elec. Nerve Stim.
90900	Biofeedback Therapy
90020	Initial Eval./Re-eval.
98000	AV-MED
97700	Worker's Comp. Assessment
97200	Hip Office Visit
97201	Hip, Add. 15 Min.
	Equipment/Ed. Supplies

_____ Other _____

( ) **Partial Bill**   ( ) **Final Bill**

DATE OF SERVICE	DESCRIPTION							TOTAL CHARGES
	CODE	AMOUNT	CODE	AMOUNT	CODE	AMOUNT	CODE	AMOUNT
1.								
2.								
3.								
4.								
5.								
6.								
7.								
8.								

TOTAL

DIAGNOSIS: _____

ASSIGNMENT AND RELEASE: I hereby authorize my insurance benefits be paid directly to Physical Therapy Institute, Inc. and I am financially responsible for non-covered services. I also authorize Physical Therapy Institute, Inc. to release any information required in the processing of this claim.

PATIENT'S SIGNATURE _____

THERAPIST'S SIGNATURE _____

T07278

Fig. 12-5. Charge slip

FORM APPROVED
OMB NO.
0938-0008

HEALTH INSURANCE CLAIM FORM
(CHECK APPLICABLE PROGRAM BLOCK BELOW)

| ☐ MEDICARE (MEDICARE NO.) | ☐ MEDICAID (MEDICAID NO.) | ☐ CHAMPUS (SPONSOR'S SSN) | ☐ CHAMPVA (VA FILE NO.) | ☐ FECA BLACK LUNG (SSN) | ☐ OTHER (CERTIFICATE SSN) |

PATIENT AND INSURED (SUBSCRIBER) INFORMATION

1. PATIENT'S NAME (LAST NAME, FIRST NAME, MIDDLE INITIAL)

2. PATIENT'S DATE OF BIRTH

3. INSURED'S NAME (LAST NAME, FIRST NAME, MIDDLE INITIAL)

4. PATIENT'S ADDRESS (STREET, CITY, STATE, ZIP CODE)

5. PATIENT'S SEX
☐ MALE ☐ FEMALE

6. INSURED'S I.D. NO. (FOR PROGRAM CHECKED ABOVE, INCLUDE ALL LETTERS)

7. PATIENT'S RELATIONSHIP TO INSURED
☐ SELF ☐ SPOUSE ☐ CHILD ☐ OTHER

8. INSURED'S GROUP NO. (OR GROUP NAME OR FECA CLAIM NO.)

TELEPHONE NO.

9. OTHER HEALTH INSURANCE COVERAGE (ENTER NAME OF POLICYHOLDER AND PLAN NAME AND ADDRESS AND POLICY OR MEDICAL ASSISTANCE NUMBER)

10. WAS CONDITION RELATED TO:
A. PATIENT'S EMPLOYMENT
☐ YES ☐ NO
B. ACCIDENT
☐ AUTO ☐ OTHER

☐ INSURED IS EMPLOYED AND CARRIED BY EMPLOYER HEALTH PLAN

11. INSURED'S ADDRESS (STREET, CITY, STATE, ZIP CODE)

TELEPHONE NO.

11.a. CHAMPUS SPONSOR'S:

| STATUS | ☐ ACTIVE DUTY ☐ RETIRED | ☐ DECEASED | BRANCH OF SERVICE |

12. PATIENT'S OR AUTHORIZED PERSON'S SIGNATURE (READ BACK BEFORE SIGNING)
I AUTHORIZE THE RELEASE OF ANY MEDICAL INFORMATION NECESSARY TO PROCESS THIS CLAIM. I ALSO REQUEST PAYMENT OF GOVERNMENT BENEFITS EITHER TO MYSELF OR TO THE PARTY WHO ACCEPTS ASSIGNMENT BELOW.

13. I AUTHORIZE PAYMENT OF MEDICAL BENEFITS TO UNDERSIGNED PHYSICIAN OR SUPPLIER FOR SERVICE DESCRIBED BELOW.

SIGNED _____ DATE _____

SIGNED (INSURED OR AUTHORIZED PERSON)

PHYSICIAN OR SUPPLIER INFORMATION

14. DATE OF: ▲ ILLNESS (FIRST SYMPTOM) OR INJURY (ACCIDENT) OR PREGNANCY (LMP)

15. DATE FIRST CONSULTED YOU FOR THIS CONDITION

16. IF PATIENT HAS HAD SAME OR SIMILAR ILLNESS OR INJURY, GIVE DATES.

16.a. IF EMERGENCY CHECK HERE ☐

17. DATE PATIENT ABLE TO RETURN TO WORK

18. DATES OF TOTAL DISABILITY
FROM _____ THROUGH _____
DATES OF PARTIAL DISABILITY
FROM _____ THROUGH _____

19. NAME OF REFERRING PHYSICIAN OR OTHER SOURCE (e.g. PUBLIC HEALTH AGENCY)

20. FOR SERVICES RELATED TO HOSPITALIZATION GIVE HOSPITALIZATION DATES
ADMITTED _____ DISCHARGED _____

184

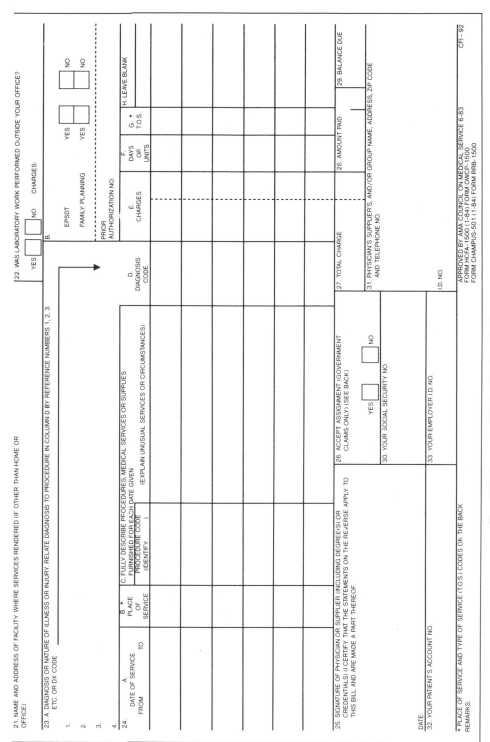

Fig. 12-6. A sample HCFA 1500 form for insurance claims.

185

familiar with its use. The ICD-9-CM may be purchased from Government Printing Office book stores or by writing or telephoning the Superintendent of Documents at the United States Government Printing Office.

Provide Charges to Office Personnel

Unless patients are charged a flat fee per visit, the therapist who treated the patient must provide the office staff with the appropriate charges for each visit. To provide a method of communication between the office staff and the therapist, a charge slip must be developed for the therapist to submit with the CPT-4 codes. These codes are procedure codes for reporting medical services and procedures performed. The slip must include all possible services and equipment for purchase. It does not have to include the actual cost of the services if the office staff has the fee schedule readily handy (Fig. 12-5).

Post Individual Patient Charges

Charges for each patient must be logged directly into the computer or onto his or her ledger card. This will provide immediate access to patient account information: specifically charges, payments, credits, and adjustments. If the billing system is not computerized, the ledger card can be photocopied and used as a monthly statement. It can be mailed to a patient when requesting payment for services.

Collect Patient Portion

The best guarantee of receiving the patient's portion of the bill is to collect the money when services are rendered. The office staff must be prepared with a current list of patients and each patient's copayment responsibility. Putting 80 percent by a specific name informs the receptionist that she must collect 20 percent of the office visit when the service is rendered. The office staff must be friendly but persistent in collecting money from the patients. Once the patient is discharged, it is less likely that payment will be received.

Produce Bills

Whether the office billing is computerized or manual, the information from the individual patient accounts must be transposed onto generic insurance forms. The HCFA 1500 forms (Fig. 12-6), used most frequently, are submitted for each patient to his or her insurance carrier. The forms must be signed by the treating therapist before submission. Certain insurance companies will not accept stamped signatures or photocopied claims for the initial submission of a claim.

Inspect Bills and Mail

Claims that are submitted with mistakes or omissions will be returned by the insurance carrier for correction. The extra time taken to review the claims for accuracy will save the time it takes to resubmit rejected claims.

ACCOUNTS RECEIVABLE AND COLLECTION PROCEDURES

When services are rendered they are either charged to the patient directly or submitted for reimbursement by third-party insurance carriers.

Collection Policies

Several options are available when collecting payment. The office can establish a policy of *payment upon services rendered,* which demands that the patient pay directly to the office. The office can then assist the patient in completing the insurance forms for submission by the patient. This policy keeps the accounts receivable to a minimum and saves the office personnel the time and trouble of dealing with insurance companies. By definition, accounts receivable are records of charges owed by patients for professional services already rendered. Most practices, particularly new ones, do not operate on such a cash-for-service basis because many patients will refuse to pay for the services directly and will take their business to another practice. Not collecting directly from the patient, however, creates a high number of outstanding accounts receivable.

A more common collection policy is to process the insurance claims as a courtesy to the patient. Immediate payment is requested for any copayment, deductible, or percentage that the insurance does not pay. This minimizes the patient's out-of-pocket expenses when the service is rendered. This is a good marketing policy for new practices, but it creates more work for the office staff and a potential cash-flow problem. An experienced office staff is required to keep the collection ratio at an acceptable level when billing the insurance companies directly.

The *collection ratio* is the total amount billed divided by the total amount collected. For example, if the office generated $10,000 of revenue and collected $7,500 of the fees billed, the collection ratio is 75 percent. A high collection ratio and a low number of aged accounts receivable characterize an effective and efficient collection procedure.

Collection Procedures

Collecting Fees From Patients

1. Collect the patient-owed portion of the bill or the entire amount at the time the service is provided.
2. Provide the patient with a signed receipt that includes the information that the patient requires to submit to the insurance company.
3. If the patient does not pay when services are provided, place a tickler on the patient's ledger card to remind the office staff to collect payment at the patient's next scheduled appointment.
4. Set up a collection timetable for overdue accounts. The most common aged-

accounts timetable is 0–30 days, 30–60 days, 60–90 days, 90–120 days, and over 120 days.

5. Set up a routine for regularly reviewing patient accounts. A common practice is to divide the accounts A–D, E–K, L–R, and S–Z. Have the office staff review and process A–D the first week of the month, E–K the second week of the month, and so forth.

6. Create standard reminder letters for accounts 30–60 days overdue and 60–90 days overdue, and a final letter sending them to collection. These standard letters can be placed on a word processor or be massed printed with blanks to be individually filled in by the office staff (Figs. 12-7 to 12-9).

a. An alternative to letters is to stamp the statements with different reminders at appropriate intervals.

7. Place all correspondence in the patient's chart and note the date on the patient's ledger card.

8. Phone inquiries are an effective way to augment the written correspondence.

9. An alternative to tracking collection letters and phone inquiries on the ledger cards is to create collection control cards on any accounts that are 30 days past due.

Collecting Fees From Insurance Companies

1. Confirm coverage and the mailing address on every patient and make sure that the standard HCFA 1500 form is acceptable.

2. Complete claims accurately and completely. Avoid any excuse for the insurance carrier to reject the claim.

3. Use the same review routine for outstanding insurance accounts.

4. Create a standard claims-status inquiry letter to be submitted to all claims not paid within 30–60 days (Fig. 12-10).

5. Initiate phone inquiries on every account 45 days past due. Document the name of the insurance clerk who confirms the status of the account.

6. Use collection control cards for accounts not reimbursed within 45 days.

7. Consider using certified mail, return receipt requested, on important correspondence with insurance carriers so that the practice has written proof that the insurance company received it.

Collection Agencies and Legal Interventions

Collection agencies and legal interventions are usually used only as a last resort. The cost, in terms of dollars and goodwill, must be considered carefully. The only accounts that should be turned over for collection are those that have had absolutely no response to normal collection efforts. Furthermore, if the account is for a small amount, it may cost more to collect than it is worth.

The collection agency should be chosen with a great deal of care as it will reflect on the practice's image. Most agencies are privately owned and operated and should be investigated to ensure selection of a reliable, ethical agency.

Although legal intervention is generally inadvisable because of the cost, time

May 25, 1989

Bill Smith
200 Lake Worth Road
Lake Worth, Florida   00000

Dear Mr. Smith:

Please be advised that there is a balance on your account
of $500.00. This balance has been in place since January
1, 1989.

Please send us full payment in the enclosed self-
addressed stamped envelop.   We will then mail you a
receipt that you can use for tax purposes or for submittal
to your secondary insurance company.

If you have any questions regarding this bill please feel
free to contact me between the hours of 10AM - 4PM Monday
through Friday.

Sincerely,

Fig. 12-7. Sample collection letter—first request for payment.

May 25, 1989

Bill Smith
200 Lake Worth Road
Lake Worth, Florida   00000

Dear Mr. Smith:

Please be advised that there is **still** a balance on your
account of $500.00. This balance has been in place since
January 1, 1989.

Please contact me immediately if you wish to discuss this
account or set up payment terms with this office. It is
imperative that we receive your payment now or
satisfactory arrangements made for taking care of your
balance due.

I shall hold your file fifteen (15) days awaiting your
reply.

Sincerely,

Fig. 12-8. Sample collection letter—second request.

May 25, 1989

Bill Smith
200 Lake Worth Road
Lake Worth, Florida   00000

Dear Mr. Smith:

Repeated requests for payment of your past due account
have been ignored.

Unless the amount of $500.00 is paid in Cash or Cashier's
check within ten (10) days from the date of this notice,
your account will be turned over to an outside collection
agency or taken to Small Claims Court.

Sincerely,

Fig. 12-9. Sample collection letter—final request before sending to a collection agency.

taken away from patients, and the loss of goodwill, there are circumstances that justify it. In many states, physical therapists can use the Small Claims Court as the legal arena, at a nominal fee.

Several factors should be considered when deciding on whether to pursue legal action. They are as follows: (1) all other avenues have been exhausted, (2) the amount outstanding is substantial, (3) the patient's ability to pay, (4) substantiation that the fees charged were appropriate, and (5) supporting documentation is indisputable.

Troubleshooting Collection Flaws

If an account receivable is never collected it is usually because of inadequate in-office procedures in one or more of five areas:

1. Office staff should strongly encourage patients to pay their office charges as they leave the office instead of being billed by mail.
2. Overdue accounts should be identified by other than general ledger cards. Easy access to the accounts receivable is essential for accurate follow-up.
3. Standardize collection notification procedures. Patients who have overdue accounts should be notified at specified intervals and with professionally written letters.
4. Personal contact will maximize office-patient relations. This requires a

```
┌─────────────────────────────────────────────────────────────┐
│              INSURANCE CLAIM STATUS REQUEST                   │
│                                                              │
│  POLICY # _____    DATE _____       │
│                                                              │
│  INSURED'S                                                   │
│  NAME _____        │
│                                                              │
│  ADDRESS _____       │
│                                                              │
│         _____      │
│                                                              │
│  PATIENT'S                      RELATIONSHIP                  │
│  NAME _____        TO INSURED _____      │
│                                                              │
│      CLAIM FOR PROFESSIONAL SERVICES WAS SUBMITTED ON         │
│                                                              │
│      _____       │
│                                                              │
│  Please indicate the status of this claim below and return   │
│  to this office.                                             │
│                                                              │
│     ___ Claim still pending because _____        │
│                                                              │
│     ___ Payment of claim in process; expected completion     │
│         date is _____                            │
│                                                              │
│     ___ Benefits in the amount of $ _____ paid to        │
│         policy holder on _____                   │
│                                                              │
│     ___ No benefits payable.                                 │
│                                                              │
│         SIGNED _____       │
│                                                              │
│         INS. CO. _____       │
│                                                              │
│         CLAIM # _____    DATE _____       │
└─────────────────────────────────────────────────────────────┘
```

Fig. 12-10. Insurance claim status request form.

well-rehearsed office person to contact by phone the patient in question and work out a financial solution to the overdue account.
5. Consider accepting credit cards as a method of collection if the demographics of the patient population justify the expense.

SUMMARY

The challenge of collecting payment in a professional and timely manner is formidable. The key to success is to maintain an organized office and to stay on top of each situation. Modification and review of the existing system and flaws as they are detected will keep the outstanding accounts receivable at an acceptable level and cash flow at an optimal level.

SUGGESTED READINGS

Beck LC: Can a pegboard really outwork a computer? Medical Economics, p. 125, December 21, 1987

ICD-9-CM Series. Superintendent of Documents, United States Government Printing Office, Washington, DC 20202

Owens A: Should you let patients pay with credit cards? Medical Economics, p. 209, March 16, 1987

Soukhanov AH: Webster's Medical Office Handbook. G. & C. Merriam Co., Philippines, 1979

Wiley MJ: Make an office computer earn its keep. Medical Economics, p. 140, August 10, 1987

Ziegler AB: Billing and Collections. Medical Economics Books, Oradel, NJ, 1979

Zupko KA: What to do about overdue accounts. Medical Economics, p. 219, March 17, 1986

APPENDIX 12-1

MEDICARE INTEMEDIARIES BY STATE

ALABAMA
Medicare Coordinator
Blue Cross and Blue Shield of
 Alabama
450 Riverchase Parkway East
Birmingham, AL 35298

ARKANSAS
Vice President for Medicare and
 Medical Services
Arkansas Blue Cross and Blue
 Shield, Inc.
601 Gaines Street
Little Rock, AR 72203

CALIFORNIA
Medicare Coordinator
California Physicians Service (d/b/a
 Blue Shield of California)
P.O. Box 7013
No. 2 Northport
San Francisco, CA 90054

Medicare Coordinator
Transamerica Occidental Life
 Insurance Company
P.O. Box 54905
Terminal Annex
Los Angeles, CA 90054

COLORADO
Assistant Vice President
Rocky Mountain Hospital and
 Medical Service (d/b/a Blue Cross
 and Blue Shield of Colorado)
700 Broadway
Denver, CO 80273

CONNECTICUT
Medicare Administrator
Travelers Insurance Company
One Tower Square
Hartford, CT 06183

Medicare Administrator
Aetna Life & Casualty
151 Farmington Avenue
Hartford, CT 06156

FLORIDA
Medicare Coordinator
Blue Cross and Blue Shield of
 Florida, Inc.
P.O. Box 1798
Jacksonville, FL 32231

ILLINOIS
Health Care Service Corporation
233 North Michigan Avenue
Chicago, IL 60601

INDIANA
Associated Insurance Companies, Inc.
 (d/b/a Blue Cross and Blue Shield
 of Indiana)
8320 Craig Street, Suite 100
Indianapolis, IN 46250-0453

IOWA
Assistant Executive Director
Blue Shield of Iowa
Ruan Building
636 Grand Avenue, Station 28
Des Moines, IO 50309

KANSAS
Medicare Assistant
Blue Cross and Blue Shield of
    Kansas, Inc.
P.O. Box 239
Topeka, KS 66601

KENTUCKY
Blue Cross and Blue Shield of
    Kentucky, Inc.
100 E. Vine Street, 6th Floor
Lexington, KY 40517

MARYLAND
Medicare Coordinator
Blue Cross and Blue Shield of
    Maryland, Inc.
700 E. Joppa Road
Baltimore, MD 21204

MASSACHUSETTS
Medicare Coordinator Part B
Blue Shield of Massachusetts, Inc.
100 Summer Street
Boston, MA 02110

MICHIGAN
Assistant Vice President
Government Affairs Department
Blue Cross and Blue Shield of
    Michigan
600 Lafayette East
Detroit, MI 48226

MINNESOTA
Blue Cross and Blue Shield of
    Minnesota
P.O. Box 64357
3535 Blue Cross Road
St. Paul, MN 55164

MISSOURI
Vice President Government Programs
Blue Cross and Blue Shield of Kansas
    City
P.O. Box 169
Kansas City, MO 64141

MISSOURI
Director of Medicare Administration
General American Life Insurance
    Company
P.O. Box 505
St. Louis, MO 63168

MONTANA
Blue Cross and Blue Shield of
    Montana, Inc.
P.O. Box 4309
Fuller Avenue
Helena, MT 59601

NEW JERSEY
Medicare Coordinator
Prudential Insurance Company of
    America
Tri-City Office Drawer 471
Millville, NJ 08332

NEW YORK
Director of Medicare Part B
Blue Shield of Western New York,
    Inc.
298 Main Street
Buffalo, NY 14202

Medicare Coordinator
Group Health Insurance, Inc.
330 West 42nd Street
New York, NY 10036

Medicare Coordinator
Empire Blue Cross and Blue Shield
622 Third Avenue
New York, NY 10019

NORTH DAKOTA
Medicare Coordinator
Blue Cross and Blue Shield of North
    Dakota
4510 13th Avenue, S.W.
Fargo, ND 58121

OHIO
Medicare System and Processing
    Division
Nationwide Mutual Insurance
    Company
P.O. Box 16788
Columbus, OH 43216

PENNSYLVANIA
Medicare Coordinator
Pennsylvania Blue Shield
P.O. Box 65
Camp Hill, PA 17011

PUERTO RICO
Chief, Internal Operations
Seguros de Servicio de Salud de
Puerto Rico, Inc.
G.P.O. Box 3628
San Juan, Puerto Rico 00936-3628

RHODE ISLAND
Medicare Coordinator
Blue Cross and Blue Shield of Rhode
Island
444 Westminster Mall
Providence, RI 02901

SOUTH CAROLINA
Medicare Coordinator
Blue Cross and Blue Shield of South
Carolina
Fontaine Business Center
300 Arbor Lake Drive, # 1300
Columbia, SC 39223

TEXAS
Blue Cross and Blue Shield of Texas,
Inc.
901 South Central Expressway
P.O. Box 833815
Richardson, TX 75083-3815

UTAH
Manager, Part B
Blue Cross and Blue Shield of Utah
P.O. Box 30270
2455 Parley's Way
Salt Lake City, UT 84130

WASHINGTON
Assistant Administrator
Washington Physicians Service
4th and Battery Building
2401 4th Avenue, 6th Floor
Seattle, WA 98121

WISCONSIN
Director, Medicare Claims
Department
Wisconsin Physicians' Service
Insurance Corp.
1717 West Broadway
Monona, WI 53713

APPENDIX 12-2

STATE WORKERS' COMPENSATION ADMINISTRATORS

ALABAMA
Workmen's Compensation Division
Dept. of Industrial Relations
Industrial Relations Building
Montgomery, AL 36130
205-261-2868

ALASKA
Division of Workers Compensation
Department of Labor
P.O. Box 1149
Juneau, AK 99802-0700
907-465-2790

ARIZONA
Industrial Commission
800 West Washington
P.O. Box 19070
Phoenix, AZ 85007
602-255-4661

ARKANSAS
Workers Compensation Commission
Justice Building
State Capitol Grounds
Little Rock, AR 72201
501-372-3930

CALIFORNIA
Division of Industrial Accidents
P.O. Box 603, Room 103
San Francisco, CA 94101
415-557-3542

COLORADO
Workers Compensation Section
Division of Labor
1313 Sherman Street, Room 314
Denver, CO 80203
303-866-2861

CONNECTICUT
Workers Compensation Commission
1890 Dixwell Avenue
Hamden, CT 06514
203-789-7783

DELAWARE
Industrial Accident Board
State Office Building, 6th Floor
820 North French Street
Wilmington, DE 19801
302-571-2885

DISTRICT OF COLUMBIA
Department of Employment Services
Office of Workers Compensation
P.O. Box 56098
Washington, DC 20011
202-576-6265

FLORIDA
Division of Workers Compensation
Department of Labor and
   Employment Security
1321 Executive Center Drive-East
Tallahassee, FL 32399-0680
904-488-2514

GEORGIA
Board of Workers Compensation
South Tower, Suite 1000
One CNN Center
Atlanta, GA 30303-2705
404-656-3875

GUAM
Workers Compensation Commission
Department of Labor
Government of Guam
P.O. Box 23548
Guam Main Facility 96921-0318

HAWAII
Disability Compensation Division
Dept. of Labor and Industrial
    Relations
830 Punchbowl Street, Room 209
Honolulu, HI 96813
808-548-4131

IDAHO
Industrial Commission
317 Main Street
Boise, ID 83720
208-334-6000

ILLINOIS
Industrial Commission
100 West Randolph Street
Suite 8-200
Chicago, IL 60601
312-917-6611

INDIANA
Industrial Board
601 State Office Building
100 North Senate Avenue
Indianapolis, IN 46204
317-232-3808

IOWA
Division of Industrial Services
Dept. of Employment Services
507 10th Street
Des Moines, IO 50319
515-281-5935

KANSAS
Division of Workers Compensation
Department of Human Resources
First Floor
217 Southeast Fourth Street
Topeka, KS 66603-3599
913-296-3441

KENTUCKY
Workers Compensation Board
127 South Building
U.S. 127 South
Frankfort, KY 40601
502-564-5550

LOUISIANA
Department of Labor
Office of Workers Compensation
    Administration
910 North Bon Marche Drive
Baton Rouge, LA 70806-2288
504-922-0158

MARYLAND
Workers Compensation Commission
6 North Liberty Street
Baltimore, MD 21201
301-659-4775

MASSACHUSETTS
Department of Industrial Accidents
100 Cambridge Street
Boston, MA 02202
617-727-3400

MICHIGAN
Bureau of Workers Disability
    Compensation
309 North Washington
Lansing, MI 48909
517-373-3480

MINNESOTA
Workers Compensation Division
Space Center, 5th Floor
444 Lafayette Road
St. Paul, MN 55101
612-296-6107

MISSISSIPPI
Workman's Compensation
  Commission
1428 Lakeland Drive
Jackson, MS 39216
601-987-4200

MISSOURI
Division of Workers Compensation
722 Jefferson Street
Jefferson City, MO 65101
314-751-4231

MONTANA
Division of Workers Compensation
Five South
Last Chance Gulch
Helena, MT 59601
406-444-6500

NEBRASKA
Workers Compensation Court
State Capital
Lincoln, NE 68509
402-471-2568

NEVADA
State Industrial Insurance System
515 East Musser Street
Carson City, NV 89714
702-885-5284

NEW HAMPSHIRE
Department of Labor
19 Pillsbury Street
Concord, NH 03301
603-271-3176

NEW JERSEY
Division of Workers Compensation
C.N. 381
Trenton, NJ 08625
609-292-2414

NEW MEXICO
Workmen's Compensation
  Administration
P.O. Box 1928
Albuquerque, NM 87103
505-841-8538

NEW YORK
Workers Compensation Board
180 Livingston Street
Brooklyn, NY 11248
718-802-6600

NORTH CAROLINA
North Carolina Industrial
  Commission
430 North Salisbury Street
Raleigh, NC 277611
919-733-4820

NORTH DAKOTA
Workmen's Compensation Bureau
Russell Building—Highway 83 North
4007 North State Street
Bismarck, ND 58501
701-224-2700

OHIO
Bureau of Workers Compensation
246 North High Street
Columbus, OH 43215
614-466-2950

OKLAHOMA
Oklahoma Workers Compensation
  Court
1915 North Stiles Street
Oklahoma City, OK 73105
405-557-7600

OREGON
Workers Compensation Department
Labor and Industries Building
Salem, OR 97310
503-378-3304

PENNSYLVANIA
Bureau of Workers Compensation
Department of Labor
3607 Derry Street
Harrisburg, PA 17111
717-783-5421

PUERTO RICO
Industrial Commissioner's Office
G.P.O. Box 446
San Juan, Puerto Rico 00936
809-783-2028

RHODE ISLAND
Dept. of Workers Compensation
610 Manton Avenue
P.O. Box 3500
Providence, RI 02909
401-272-0700

SOUTH CAROLINA
Workers Compensation Commission
1612 Marion Street
P.O. Box 1715
Columbia, SC 29202
803-737-5700

SOUTH DAKOTA
Division of Labor and Management
Department of Labor
Kneip Building, Second Floor
700 Illinois North
Pierre, SD 57501
605-773-3681

TENNESSEE
Workers Compensation Division
Department of Labor
501 Union Building
Second Floor
Nashville, TN 37219
615-741-2395

TEXAS
Industrial Accident Board
200 E. Riverside Drive, 1st Floor
Austin, TX 78704
512-448-7900

UTAH
Industrial Commission
160 East 300 South
Salt Lake City, UT 84145
801-530-6800

VERMONT
Department of Labor and Industry
120 State Street
Montpelier, VT 05602
802-828-2286

VIRGIN ISLANDS
Department of Labor
P.O. Box 450
Christiansted
St. Croix, Virgin Islands
809-773-6200

VIRGINIA
Industrial Commission
1000 DMV Building
P.O. Box 1794
Richmond, VA 23214
804-257-8600

WASHINGTON
Department of Labor and Industries
General Administration Building
AX-31
Olympia, WA 98504
206-753-6341

WEST VIRGINIA
Workers Compensation
  Commissioner's Office
P.O. Box 3151
Charleston, WV 25332
304-348-2580

WISCONSIN
Workers Compensation Division
Department of Industry, Labor and
  Human Relations
P.O. Box 7901
201 E. Washington Avenue, #161
Madison, WI 53707
608-266-1340

WYOMING
Workers Compensation Division
State Treasurer's Office
122 W. 25th Street, 2nd Floor
East Wing, Herschler Building
Cheyenne, WY 82002
307-777-7411

13

ONGOING AND FUTURE CONSIDERATIONS: LEGISLATIVE, LEGAL CONCERNS, AND EXPANSION

This chapter assumes that the private physical therapy practice is succeeding or at least surviving. As one goes through the developmental and management steps discussed in earlier chapters, the practice assumes a form all its own. The patients, the reimbursement, the performance of the employees, and other aspects will all be unique, as no two practices are exactly alike.

The most important thing to avoid when the private practice is succeeding is complacency. A private practitioner who becomes content, smug, or self-satisfied is asking for problems. The independently owned physical therapy practice is always vulnerable. A relaxed feeling about success can quickly lead to a turn in the negative direction.

There are many future concerns both short- and long-term, that must constantly be evaluated, such as changing environment, internal expansion, external expansion, office purchase, and possible sale of the practice.

CHANGING ENVIRONMENT

The health care environment is an ever-changing one, a fact that has significant impact on all health care providers, especially those in private practice. Keeping abreast of the environment on the national and local levels will allow the practice to take initiatives rather than merely to react.

Legislative Concerns

Physical therapists are licensed to practice in their respective states by state boards that oversee the profession and determine the rules and regulations under which physical therapists practice. Changes in the legislative area directly affect physical therapists.

In some states physical therapists are permitted to evaluate and treat patients without a referring physician. This direct access privilege is a result of legislative action. In some states physicians are permitted to employ physical therapist assistants without hiring physical therapists to oversee them, and in still other states occupational therapists have the right to use physical therapy treatment methods. These various situations all result from legislative change.

When legislation affecting physical therapy is before a legislative body, many professional organizations will wish to have a voice. The associations that represent physicians and chiropractors are the two primary organizations (other than the American Physical Therapy Association) that are concerned with physical therapy legislation. These organizations usually oppose legislative changes that promote independence of physical therapists. Because of the opposition of medical and chiropractic organizations, which believe it is in their interest to keep the physical therapy profession in a subordinate position, it is difficult for physical therapists to promote their profession as much as they would like.

For physical therapists to succeed in obtaining favorable legislation, they must present a united front in lobbying the legislatures. This requires effort from all physical therapists as well as financial support. Physical therapy is a smaller and less financially solvent profession than medicine and chiropractic.

Any legislative change in medical policies that is not in the interest of physical therapy usually hurts the profession. Therefore, private physical therapists must take a very active role in the legislative efforts of their professional association. Being aware of proposed legislative changes before they occur is the way to stop some adverse changes. Additionally, if legislation damaging to the practice of physical therapy is passed, private practitioners need to know in advance to make the necessary adjustments for the continued success of their practice.

Insurance Reimbursement

The issue of insurance reimbursement is related to that of legislation. Changes in reimbursement policies have a considerable impact on health care providers; most such changes have worked to the disadvantage of the private physical therapist. Two areas of major concern are Medicare and Workers' Compensation.

Medicare is a federally funded program and therefore falls under federal guidelines. Presently, Medicare reimbursements for outpatient physical therapy services are low. However, patients who receive physical therapy in a hospital, a certified rehabilitation agency, or a physician's office fall under different guidelines. This inequity can only be challenged, and hopefully changed, at the federal level. Meanwhile, private physical therapy practices have a serious problem concerning the Medicare population. If the practice accepts Medicare assignment, how are these patients to be charged after the Medicare limit is reached? Should the practice not accept Medicare patients and thereby risk the loss of referral sources who treat such patients? This issue must be decided in a way that proves profitable for the private practice.

Workers' Compensation is a state-funded program and therefore falls under state guidelines. Therefore, the guidelines for Workers' Compensation vary from state to state. The Workers' Compensation board for the state periodically reviews past charges for specific health services and then selects a percentile of the charges as a basis for the new fee schedule. The schedule selected on the basis of prior charges does not take into consideration the different types of facilities providing the services and is generally lower than the practice's usual and customary fees. Therefore, Workers' Compensation patients are another group for whom the practice is usually paid less per treatment than the standard fee. As with all regulations, there are methods to alter the situation. If the facility becomes a rehabilitation provider within the state, services are reimbursed on a higher schedule. Once again, the private physical therapy practitioner has to decide if providing therapy to a class of patients is favorable to the short- and long-term growth of the private practice.

Insurance reimbursement is a rapidly changing area, which has a clear impact on physical therapy providers and which must continually be watched and evaluated to maintain a solvent practice.

Physician–Physical Therapist Arrangements

Physician–physical therapist arrangements are growing nationally by leaps and bounds. Regardless of the legal mechanism of these endeavors, they run counter to the principles of free enterprise. Therefore, physical therapists who own private practices must keep abreast of changes in their own and adjacent communities. It is quite common when such an arrangement develops in the community for the physical therapist-owned practice to lose referral sources. Depending on the diversity of available referral sources, the impact can be disastrous. For example, if two orthopedic surgeons who formerly referred patients to the practice opened a physician-owned physical therapy service (POPTS), the practice would lose two referral sources. If these two physicians had provided 50 percent of the practice's referrals, a 50 percent drop in referrals would result; if they had referred only 20 percent of the patients, the loss would be only 20 percent. Although these sources of future referrals have been lost, the practice's costs, fixed and variable, remain the same. Therefore, this type of situation can devastate the practice, sometimes practically overnight.

This is a situation in which a complacent attitude is detrimental. If the practice is flourishing and the owners have not kept up with the changing environment, the practice can receive a major blow. However, if the owners constantly seek and obtain new referral sources, the effect is not as great. Constant solicitation of referral sources helps to keep the percentage of referrals from any source at a minimum. Additionally, the practice will benefit from the extra referrals from new sources before present sources are lost.

New Private Physical Therapy Practices

In any profession there is always competition. It is common for new physical therapy practices to open in the community. These new practices will strive to develop a referral base, thereby cutting into the market share of existing practices.

The practice cannot afford to get complacent or fail to live up to the high standards it marketed. In fact a private practice functioning at the highest level may serve to deter new private practices from opening in the same community. If the practice does get complacent it may lose some of the referral sources to the new physical therapy practices. Accordingly, no matter how successful the private practice becomes one must always maintain that eagerness to succeed.

Health Maintenance and Preferred Provider Organizations

With the impetus in society toward cost-effective health care, health maintenance organizations (HMO's) and preferred provider organizations (PPO's) are proliferating rapidly. These organizations provide health care coverage for their clients under a system designed to control costs by contracting with health care providers at fixed or reduced reimbursement schedules. As a result, the number of providers who serve the clients of these organizations is restricted. Frequently, they limit the number of physical therapy providers with whom they contract in each community.

The impact of these organizations on the physical therapy practice is that the practice secures a referral source if and only if it contracts with the organization for a reduced fee. HMOs usually develop a fixed rate of physical therapy reimbursement; PPO's generally agree to pay a percentage of the usual and customary fees. As these organizations continue to grow and to sign up clients, one must decide if the reduced rate of reimbursement is worthwhile.

Medicolegal Implications

Our health care system every day is becoming increasingly intertwined with our legal system. It is almost impossible for private physical therapy practices to avoid becoming involved in medicolegal problems, which occurs most commonly when they provide services to patients who are involved in legal action as a result, for example, of injuries received in a fall on private property or in an automobile accident.

Patients who have retained an attorney frequently request that all bills for services rendered be sent to the attorney. These patients are in the process of suing someone as a result of their injury. The practice must secure a signed medical lien, where applicable (check respective state requirements). A medical lien is a legal statement from the patient's attorney stating that after the case is resolved, the attorney will pay the bill out of the settlement (see also Ch. 12).

Furthermore, the practice must expect to receive a subpoena or a request for records from the attorney representing the patient. This subpoena or request for records usually require copies of the patient's medical records, but before these can be transmitted, the patient must have signed a release of records form, which is sent with the subpoena by the attorney. The subpoena should also be accompanied by a check for a nominal amount to cover the cost of copying and mailing the records to the attorney. The procedure for the request of records may vary from state to state.

Sometimes the attorney will want the physical therapist not only to supply the records but also to give a deposition. This is a legal statement made under oath and recorded by a court stenographer, in answer to questions from lawyers for both sides about the patient. The transcript of this deposition together with those made by other involved parties, will help the attorneys to decide whether to settle out of court or go to trial. The deposition may take anywhere from minutes to hours. It may be made in the office of one of the attorneys or even in the office of the practice. Giving depositions takes time from the regular office functions; however, the therapist should charge for the deposition and travel time. Fees for depositions vary, and one should check the usual rate with colleagues in the community.

A therapist who gives factual information about a patient is acting as a fact witness. This is the most common situation in which therapists give testimony. They may also testify as defendants if they are named in a lawsuit, usually by a patient.

Physical therapists as well as other health care providers are named as defendants usually in cases where the patient claims the provider or providers were negligent. Negligence usually comprises four elements: a duty to act, a breach of the standard of care, a breach of care causing something to happen, and a causative factor leading to harm to the patient. A therapist named as a defendant in a lawsuit must immediately contact his or her insurance company. The therapist and the insurance company then find an attorney. The defense in a negligence case is usually to prove that the therapist acted within the accepted standard of care and did what any other physical therapist in the community would have done. As more and more medicolegal claims are being settled without trial, more people are bringing suit against professionals with whom they become disenchanted. Therefore an increasing number of lawsuits are being brought against physical therapists, most of whom are private practitioners. The only way to defend a physical therapist or any health care professional is through the medical records. Strong documentation is the only basis for a strong defense.

A third way in which a physical therapist can become involved with the medicolegal system is as an expert witness. This situation usually arises when the therapist is questioned about the standard of care provided by another physical therapist. The therapist performing this service charges a fee for the review of records, meetings, travel, and testimony.

A therapist entering private practice must expect involvement in medicolegal situations, hopefully only as the supplier of patient records or as a factual witness. Although such demands disrupt the practice, they must be complied with if the therapist wishes to treat patients who have elected to use the available legal system.

Day-to-Day Impact

The changing environment has an impact on the daily functioning of the private practice. When the law changes, the private practice can change its policies accordingly. When direct access becomes available, the practice may solicit the consumer directly. When Medicare or Workers' Compensation requires additional paperwork before paying the bills for services rendered, the private practice must comply. When clinics operated by a physician–physical therapist arrangement or new private practices open, the practice must adapt to meet these challenges.

Moreover, every facet of the practice is modified on a daily basis in response to many variables. If one employee calls in sick or is on vacation, the owner must have a plan of coverage. If the practice has a computer problem and falls behind in billing and collecting revenues, there must be a contingency plan. If the three largest referral sources always take vacation during August, there must be a plan to accommodate this circumstance. To have a smooth and efficient operation the practice must have a pulse on every variable. Through this heightened awareness the private practice can be managed in a forward-looking manner instead of reacting to changes after the fact.

INTERNAL EXPANSION

As the private practice grows, the question of internal expansion (i.e., increase in staff, equipment, and space) arises continually. At some point there will be a need to hire additional staff, but the timing of such increases is a difficult decision. At which point is the work load too much for the present staff? There is no right or wrong answer to this question; however, the decision to hire additional staff should not be delayed until the practice begins to suffer. Too long a wait may cause the quality of patient care to decline, and furthermore the staff may fall behind in administrative tasks such as billing and collecting accounts receivable. Delays in tasks such as typing letters to physicians may adversely affect future referrals. One must decide when the professional staff people are unable to competently treat any more patients than they have on their roster. If the staff is overburdened, rapport with the patients may suffer. If patients are placed on a waiting list, both patients and referral sources may be lost.

However, if one chooses to hire additional employees, operating costs increase sooner than revenues. For example, if one decides to hire an additional physical therapist full-time, one must pay the physical therapist's salary and all other benefits from the day this new employee starts work. For a full-time physical therapist, the monthly cost may be assumed to be $3,000.00 It may take weeks or months before this physical therapist handles enough patients to generate $3,000 in receivables. The first $3,000 per month in added revenue only offsets the additional cost of the new employee. The additional patient load that generates revenues above $3,000 is the profit to the private practice. However, this profit margin may take months to develop, and in the interim the private practice has increased expenses without increased revenues. When hiring an administrative employee, the practice hopes to improve the administrative flow and promote maximum efficiency. Here the increased revenues result from improved efficiency, as administrative staff persons are not treating patients and producing revenues directly.

As the private practice grows, it may become apparent that additional equipment is needed. This is an increased expense whether the equipment is purchased, leased, or rented. If equipment is required to provide the quality of care promised, it is essential even though it may not appear to increase revenues. If equipment is required to develop and market a new program that results in new patients, then this equipment generates increased revenues.

If the practice is successful, it may grow beyond its physical capabilities. This leads the owners to the difficult question of whether the space should be increased. If adjacent office space is available or if a larger area is available in the building, increasing the size of the office is an option, but the costs associated with this are high. Adding the adjacent space increases the rent; moreover, any structural changes to accommodate the merging of space is usually charged to the practice. Additional costs are those for floor and wall coverings, telephones, electricity, and equipment purchases. If adjacent space is not available, then moving to a larger space is even more costly, as it is equivalent to designing and developing a new physical facility (see Ch. 6). Either way, expansion is expensive. If the expansion is extensive enough, it may require financing (see Ch. 3). However, if the private practice grows to the point that expansion is necessary, then by all means this should be considered a sign of success.

A healthy and prospering private practice must undergo internal expansion. When expanding by acquiring additional employees, equipment, or space, it must be remembered that increased costs are part of the package. There are usually delays in recouping the increased costs, but this is par for the expansion.

EXTERNAL EXPANSION

Another mode of expansion for a successful private practice is external, which essentially means development of additional private practices by opening one or more additional offices. The decision to develop an additional office in the same community may be a result of physical limitations; the practice would then be opening a second office that maintains the same standards.

The decision to develop an additional office or offices outside the community represents a different attitude toward expansion. In fact, there are companies that own facilities in many different states. This approach to expansion is based, not on supervision of more than one facility by the same respected, community-minded physical therapist, but on the increased efficiency achievable with a uniform system for servicing many clinics (e.g., centralized billing procedures, decreased equipment and supply costs through volume purchases, and decreased insurance costs due to the lower rates available to larger organizations). Additionally, companies that choose this mode of expansion strive to have physical therapists from the local communities run the respective practices, as this facilitates local community acceptance.

Regardless of the philosophy underlying the decision to open additional offices, each office must be considered as a new entity. Therefore, all the steps discussed in the preceding chapters for starting a new practice must be considered for the development and success of the new office.

One major advantage of opening a second office is the ability to obtain financing, for which the record of the first office paves the way. Tax returns for previous years and the practice's balance sheets prove that the owner has successfully built a private practice. This record of success provides greater leverage when requesting funds, so that the loan can be negotiated on more favorable terms (e.g., interest rate, fixed or variable, number of years).

One major fact to remember about starting the second office is that it takes hard work. Since the practitioner already knows how to start and run a private practice, it is natural to assume that the second office is easier; however, the second office requires as much effort and perseverance as the first, as it will most likely present a new set of issues and concerns. If one has successfully developed a private practice and decides to develop a second, the prior knowledge will definitely prove helpful, but it should not be assumed that the second office will require any less effort than the first.

Purchase of An Office

Rent is probably the highest monthly expense, and its payment provides essentially no other benefit to the practice. Therefore, a private practitioner who has become successful may consider owning office space, which allows increased tax deductions as well as building up equity.

The relationship between an owned office and the corporation is similar to that between a house and the homeowner. Instead of paying rent to a landlord, the practice pays a mortgage to a lending institution, so that the rental dollar equivalent works for the practice rather than for a landlord. Additionally, office improvements can increase the value of the office. For example, attractive cabinets built into the office usually stay with the owners of the practice, whereas in the case of rental property, these cabinets belong to the landlord if the practice is moved. Cabinets that are built into the practice's office may increase the resale value. Additionally, the depreciation allowance decreases the private practice's tax liability.

Buying an office, like buying a house, requires a down payment. In addition, financing must be found for the purchase, but this should not be too difficult, as the office serves as collateral, which protects the lender in the event that the practice defaults on the loan payments. The down payment is another problem; a large one may be required depending upon the percentage of financing.

To find office space for sale, just as to find a house for sale, one can contact a commercial realtor or check the classified ads in the newspapers. The resources of the accountant and the attorney should be used when seeking to purchase an office.

The office space may be acquired by different types of purchase; most commonly, either an office condominium or an entire office building is bought. The condominium arrangement would mean ownership of one office in a commercial office complex. This gives the practice the benefit of ownership while having all the common services provided by the condominium management. In addition to mortgage payments, the practice will have to pay a fee for the services provided to all the tenants.

The purchase of an office building can be of much greater complexity. The practitioners may purchase a whole building of appropriate square footage only for provision of physical therapy services, or they may choose to purchase a building for the physical therapy services that includes other offices for rent. In both cases one obtains the benefits, while assuming all the responsibilities, of building ownership; in the latter case one additionally assumes the responsibilities of a landlord.

If the private practice owns a building in which it occupies one of the offices, the other tenants' rent payments may pay a portion of the rent for the practice's office space, so that the owners of the practice have a form of rent-free or rent-reduced office space while still increasing their equity in the building. In practical situations a new corporation may be established to own the building, which then rents office space to the private practice and the other tenants. Even if finances are not an issue, an office building may prove to be a major source of problems to owners who are physical therapists, not office landlords. The necessary support systems should be used during this undertaking.

As landlords the owners will also have problems involving tenant complaints when things in the building are not functioning properly. It is up to the owners to solve the problems; however, they may wish to hire a building manager to deal with the complaints. Furthermore, the need for an attorney's services will be increased considerably, as the owners will be negotiating leases with the tenants.

If the private practice grows to the point that the owners are able to purchase a building, they must be doing something right. However, since owning and operating a building is a new business, totally unlike physical therapy, the owners may not be qualified to manage the building or its tenants without qualified support personnel. Support systems should be used to ensure success in this new endeavor.

SELLING THE PRACTICE

There are two primary reasons for selling a successful private practice: the owners have had enough enjoyment from their efforts and wish to change professional direction or retire; or a larger corporation desires to buy the practice. For whichever reason the question arises, one must be able to place a value on the practice to sell it.

When considering sale of a private practice, one must remember that it is a business decision and avoid being swayed by personal attachment to the practice. Additionally, the physical therapist—owner, who is probably selling a practice for the first time must realize that this type of business decision is more sophisticated than the normal day-to-day decisions. Therefore, it is imperative to rely heavily on the accountant and attorney when undertaking a sale.

There is no right way to determine the value of a private physical therapy practice. Some of the factors to consider in arriving at the right selling price are the balance sheet, income statement, tax returns, previous earnings, accounts receivable, equipment, inventory, leases, prepaid expenses, real estate and building, goodwill, and public image.

Balance Sheet

The balance sheet provides a financial summary of what the business owns and owes. The liabilities are subtracted from the assets to find the owner's equity (also called the net worth or book value). This amount is frequently used to determine the value of the private practice.

Income Statement

The income statement lists by line item for a specified period the sources of income, the sources of expenses, and the profit that the private practice is making. When the expenses of the business are subtracted from the income, the profit can be determined. Taxes are among the items that must be subtracted from the gross income to accurately assess net income. The income statements usually show the income and expenses for the specified time frame along with year-to-date totals, thus giving a clear picture of the practice's annual performance.

Tax Returns

A review of the practice's tax returns for the last few years provides an assessment of the business. If the private practice shows increased profits each year, a positive projection may be made but if its profits have declined steadily, the prospective buyer will make a less than positive projection. The former situation implies that the practice is still growing, whereas the latter situation implies that the practice is steadily declining and the owner may, in fact, be bailing out.

Previous Earnings

Previous earnings demonstrate that the private practice has earned profits. Records of previous earnings are provided by the balance sheet, income statement, and prior tax returns.

Accounts Receivable

Accounts receivable are the amounts owed to the private practice for services rendered. That clients owe money to the practice is a healthy sign, but if the dollar amounts owed become too high, this may indicate that the practice has a problem with collecting the funds due. This problem may decrease the value of the private practice because the longer any account is past due, the less the likelihood of collecting. Usually, accounts receivable are classified as 0 to 30 days, 30 to 60 days, 60 to 90 days, 90 to 120 days, and 120 days and over. When a private practice is sold, the accounts receivable can be negotiated as part of the sale. The purchaser of the practice either may allow the present owner to continue to collect the outstanding funds or may buy the outstanding funds at a discounted rate.

Equipment

If the private practice is fully equipped, the equipment may prove to be one of the largest assets in the sale. The value of the equipment is usually considered to be the price originally paid less depreciation. However, if the equipment was leased or is collateral for an outstanding loan, this must be considered in determining its value.

Inventory

Inventory, like equipment, is considered an asset. Inventory may include salable supplies, which can be turned into a profit by the new owner, and nonsalable supplies, which are supplies required to permit the practice to function effectively.

Leases

A current lease for the office may prove to be an asset when the owner desires to sell the practice. The new owner may be able to take over the lease, thereby securing office space for the newly purchased practice without having to move it. In some cases the landlord may permit transfer of the lease without any escalation and allow inclusion of all renewal options.

Prepaid Expenses

Prepaid expenses are those paid before the due date; therefore they are considered assets. Maintenance contracts on major equipment, insurance premiums, and loan installments are but a few of the items that may be prepaid. If some items are prepaid, the seller will wish to receive payment for them at the time of sale.

Real Estate and Building

Ownership of a building or even an office condominium gives the practitioner a major asset. The sale of the building or office should usually be considered as separate transactions: however, sale of the building or condominium along with the practice may be accomplished in a single transaction. When attempting to value the real estate holdings, the accountant's assistance must be secured. It should be kept in mind that the private practice can be sold and the practitioner still retain ownership of the real estate. If only the practice is sold, the new owner must rent the office space from the prior owner, who is now the landlord.

Goodwill and Public Image

Goodwill is a variable asset that the present owners and employees bring to the practice. This asset in some manner enhances desirability of the practice in the eyes of would-be purchasers. Goodwill cannot be defined as a tangible asset. An example of goodwill would be the good reputations of the clinicians in the practice, without which the value of the practice would be considerably less. Therefore, the name of the practice and the reputations of the clinicians are part of what the new owners are purchasing. If the new owners are to benefit from the intangible assets of the present practice, a dollar value must be placed on goodwill. There are no simple methods to calculate goodwill, so the buyer and seller must develop their own method. Frequently when a private practice is sold, the present owners agree to work for and thereby assist the new owners for a few years, thus providing a slow transition of ownership. Additionally, this arrangement allows the practice to continue along the same course without traumatic disruptions. While working for the new owners, the former owner is paid a salary or a consultation fee in addition to the revenues received from the sale of the practice.

Selling the private practice may prove to be a very emotional decision; however, for personal, professional, and business reasons, there may come a time when it becomes the right choice. If the practice has been successful, the seller walks away from the sale with great pride and considerable money. This is a reward for successfully building a private practice.

SUMMARY

This chapter covers some ongoing and future considerations relating to a successful private physical therapy practice. The changing health care environment is discussed in relation to legislative concerns, insurance reimbursement, physician–physical therapist arrangements, new private physical therapy practices, HMOs and PPOs, and medicolegal implications. Other topics discussed are internal and external expansion; the possibility of purchasing an office in connection with growth of the practice; and the sale of a practice for financial reward. These are but a few of the many ongoing and future planning considerations that go along with owning a physical therapy practice.

SUGGESTED READINGS

Butler KG (ed): Prospering In Private-Practice—A Handbook For Speech-Language Pathology and Audiology. Aspen Publications, Rockville, MD, 1986

Brimer MA: Fundamentals Of Private Practice In Physical Therapy. Charles C Thomas, Springfield, IL, 1988

Coughlan WD: Change and its impact on private practice physical therapists. Whirlpool 10(4):22–23, 1987

Griffith CC, Griffith C: Law for the physical therapist. Part I. Clin Management 1(4):22–24, 1981

Griffith CC, Griffith C: Law for the Physicial Therapist—Part II. Clin Management 2(1):9–10, 1982

Horting M: HMO's and the physical therapist: A growing relationship. Clin Management 7(6):30–35, 1987

Miles RC: How To Price A Business—A Guide For Buyers And Sellers. Institute for Business Planning, Englewood Cliffs, NJ, 1987

Scanlon J: Malpractice—Do you know how to protect yourself? Today's Student PT:15–19, Spring 1987

INDEX

Note: Page numbers followed by f designate figures and those followed by t designate tables.